DENTAL ASSISTING
Instrument
Guide

Second Edition

DENTAL ASSISTING
Instrument
Guide

Second Edition

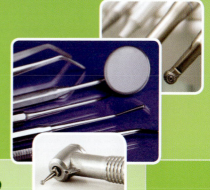

DONNA PHINNEY
CDA, BA, M.Ed
Spokane Community
College

JUDY HALSTEAD
CDA, BA
Professor Emeritus Spokane
Community College

CENGAGE Learning®

Australia • Brazil • Japan • Korea • Mexico • Singapore • Spain • United Kingdom • United States

Contents

Contents

Preface

Dental instruments are continually developing as technology changes and dental materials require instruments of specific designs or materials. Most instruments are constructed of stainless steel, and a few are a high-tech plastic/resin or anodized aluminum. Manufacturers of dental instruments provide many designs and sizes and make improvements as new materials become available. Dentists select the instruments they feel the most confident and comfortable using. Each procedure requires special instruments to accomplish the task.

For example, when examining the pits and grooves of the teeth, the dentist uses an explorer. The ends of all explorers are pointed and sharp, but they are designed with different angles to reach all surfaces of the tooth.

The dental assistant is responsible for keeping the instruments sterilized and in working condition. The dental assistant orders new instruments as needed, keeps the instruments in sequence while assisting during the procedure, and performs maintenance.

The *Dental Assisting Instrument Guide*, Second Edition is designed to give the dental

We feel students will find this guide to be a very helpful tool in their learning process as an adjunct to their main textbook and clinic/laboratory experience.

New to This Edition

Updates have been made throughout the text to address changes in instruments and equipment.

Chapter 1
- Some content has been combined where appropriate

Chapter 2
- New chapter; covers disposable equipment and barrier devices

Chapter 3
- Formerly Chapter 2

assistant the basic knowledge necessary in relationship to each instrument presented. It allows the student to view each instrument and learn its uses, parts, and other miscellaneous information. It also allows the student to test recall of each instrument and its use. The instruments are categorized in groupings that follow basic dental procedures. For example, one section covers instruments used in restorative procedures; another section covers all of the dental burs. This allows students to easily study similar information. The guide also covers sterilizing equipment and monitors. Note that additional equipment that pertains to the specific dental procedures and specialties is included, such as an endodontic electronic pulp tester, air abrasion unit, and curing lights.

- Added coverage of the following: evacuator screens, air-water syringe, Isolite system, self-contained water unit, and water line treatments

Chapter 4
- Formerly Chapter 3
- Added coverage of Jenker needlestick protector
- Updated images

Chapter 5
- Formerly Chapter 4
- Added Quick and Instant Dental Dam and Added pictures

Chapter 6
- Formerly Chapter 5
- Added information on dental units
- Updated and added pictures

Chapter 7
- Formerly Chapter 6
- Merged some content where appropriate
- Added information on the diamond turbo or speed cut and the diamond composite finishing bur
- Added drawings and pictures

Chapter 8
- Formerly Chapter 7

Chapter 9
- Formerly Chapter 8
- Added coverage of diagnostic aids: intraoral camera, cavity detection/DIAGNOdent
- Updated pictures

Chapter 10
- Formerly Chapter 9
- Updated and added pictures
- Omitted the Frahm carver

Chapter 11
- Formerly Chapter 10
- Added information on composite shade guides and composite polishers
- Updated and added pictures

Chapter 12
- Formerly Chapter 11
- Combined material on some instruments where appropriate
- Updated and added pictures

Chapter 13
- Formerly Chapter 12
- Combined content where appropriate

- Added coverage of suture scissors, root tip picks, and tray setup for suture removal
- Omitted discussion of mouth props, mouth gag.

Chapter 14
- Formerly Chapter 13
- Combined content where appropriate
- Added information on various kinds of separators
- Added coverage of Orthodontic Lip and Cheek Retractors and Self-Ligating Bracket System and Placement Instrument (Damon)

Chapter 15
- Formerly Chapter 14
- Added information on tray setup for application of dental sealants

Chapter 16
- Formerly Chapter 15
- Combined discussion of some instruments where appropriate
- Updated and added pictures
- Omitted the implant scaler,

Chapter 17
- Formerly Chapter 16
- Added discussion of computer-aided design (CAD) and computer-aided manufacturing (CAM)
- Content on implants moved to Chapter 18
- Omitted wooden bite stick and shade guide information

Chapter 18
- New chapter focusing on implant systems; content was formerly combined with Chapter 16
- Former Chapter 17 has been omitted.

Chapter 19
- Formerly Chapter 18
- Sterilization information is updated

Chapter 20
- New chapter focusing on laboratory equipment

Chapter 21
- New chapter focusing on radiology equipment

Acknowledgments

We want to thank those who encouraged and motivated us to develop this instrument guide. Thanks to our students for asking us to develop better ways to learn and remember instruments that are used in dental procedures. Each year, students' quest for knowledge becomes more creative and inventive. A quick reference is necessary in the busy lives of students who must fit so many things into their schedules. Our goal was a quick reference to meet their needs.

Next we thank Hu-Friedy and Miltex for their photos and cooperation. Both of these companies as well as many others aided us with this project. A special thank-you goes to Mike Galatelli, photographer, for his eye for design and detail and his talent in obtaining the photos for this pocket guide.

We would like to thank Cengage Learning and its staff, whose assistance and encouragement in this project are greatly appreciated. We would like to especially acknowledge Tari Broderick, Acquisitions Editor, for continuing support and leadership, and Darcy Scelsi, Senior Product Manager, for her dedication and guidance with this project and her organization and keen eye during the photo shoot.

Last, but never least, we would like to thank our husbands, Dwayne and Chuck, and our families, for their continued support throughout all of our endeavors.

Description of Icons

Heat Sterilization   Cold Sterilization   Disposable

Disinfect   Sharps Container

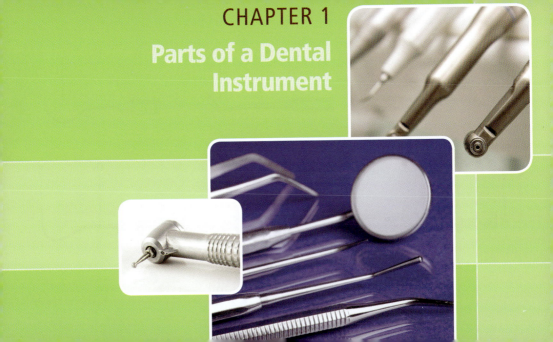

CHAPTER 1

Parts of a Dental Instrument

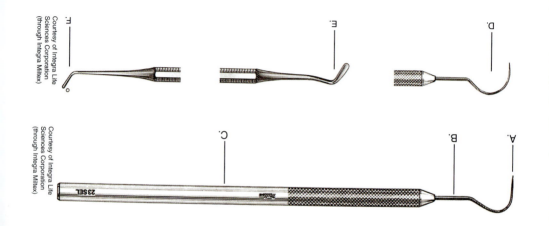

F.

E.

D.

C.

B.

A.

Basic Structural Parts and Working Ends of Dental Instruments

Use

Dental instruments are used to accomplish a variety of tasks. Each procedure requires special instruments for its unique tasks. Most instruments are constructed of stainless steel, high-tech plastic/resin, or anodized aluminum. The working end of an instrument performs the specific function of the instrument.

Parts

A. Working end
B. Shank
C. Handle

The working end may be a point, blade, or nib.

D. The point is sharp and is used to explore, detect, and reflect materials.
E. The blade may be flat or curved and may have a rounded or cutting edge.
F. The nib is a blunt end that may be serrated or smooth.

Misc.

There are single- and double-ended instruments. On some double-ended instruments the primary working end is marked with an indented ring around the shank or the handle.

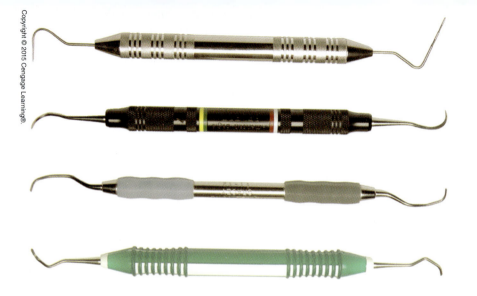

Ergonomically Designed Handles

Use

The handle or shaft of an instrument is where the instrument is held by the operator. Some handles are ergonomically designed for easier handling and better grip.

Misc.

- In traditional instruments, handles may be smooth, serrated, round, or hexagonal (six sided). Some may have cone socket handles that allow the working ends to be replaced.
- Ergonomic handles may be larger and designed with rests and grooves.
- Some handles are covered with a soft, rubber-like material for more comfortable handling.
- Handles are made of lightweight, sterilizible materials.

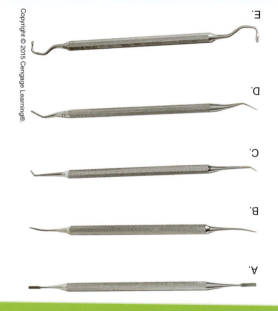

E.

D.

C.

B.

A.

The Shank

Use

The shank connects the handle to the working end. It narrows or tapers from the handle to the working end. The shank may be angled to reach different areas of the mouth. Instruments that are used in the posterior regions of the mouth have more angles, whereas straighter or slightly curved instruments are used in the anterior regions.

Types

A. Straight (no angles)
B. Curved (slightly curved)
C. Monangle (one angle)
D. Binangle (two angles)
E. Triple angle (three angles)

A.

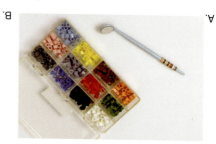

B.

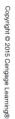 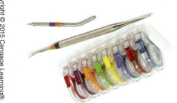

C.

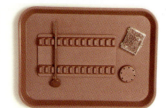

Use

Color coding is a method used to easily identify instruments, tubs, and trays. Color coding may be used to indicate the sequence of a procedure, additional sets of instruments, treatment rooms where instruments are stored, individual operators, or any combination of these.

Parts

There are many types of materials used for color coding, including:

A. Plastic rings

B. Tape

C. Color-coded tray, mouth mirror, bur block, tray mat, and plastic rings (Color-coded tubs and various-size trays are also available.)

Misc.

Materials used for color coding must be autoclavable and durable.

Test Your Knowledge

_____ 1. This part of a dental instrument may be a point, blade, or nib.
   A. Handle
   B. Shank
   C. Working end

_____ 2. This part of a dental instrument may be straight, curved, monangle, binangle, or triple angle.
   A. Handle
   B. Shank
   C. Working end

_____ 3. This part of a dental instrument may be ergonomically designed.
   A. Handle
   B. Shank
   C. Working end

_____ 4. This part of a dental instrument may be smooth or serrated.

    A. Handle

    B. Shank

    C. Working end

_____ 5. This part of a dental instrument may be angled to reach different areas of the mouth.

    A. Handle

    B. Shank

    C. Working end

CHAPTER 2

Disposables and Barriers

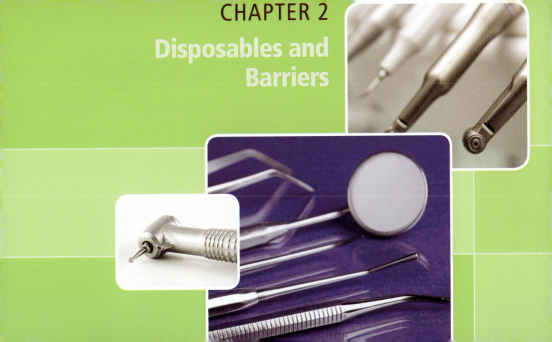

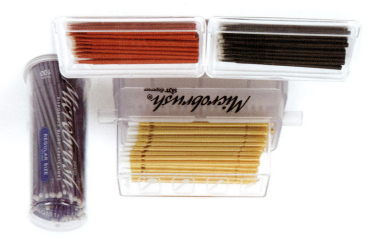

Micro Applicator and Brushes

Use	- To place etchants
	- To place bonding agents
	- To apply primer into post holes and small preps
	- To apply sealants
	- To apply cavity liners and varnishes
	- To apply hemostatic solutions
	- To get into those hard-to-reach areas
Parts	Plastic handles with micro ball end of nonabsorbent fiber or bristled tip brushes
Misc.	- Normally comes with bendable neck to allow easy placement and precise application
	- Micro applicators and brush tips available in super fine, fine, or regular/standard
	- Micro applicators and brushes available in a variety of styles, sizes, and colors
	- Both are disposable, and the brushes are available with reusable handles that fit with disposable brushes.

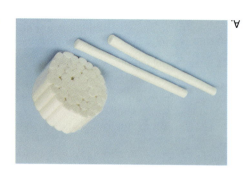

B.

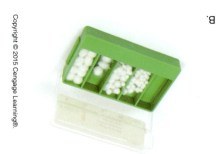

A.

Cotton Rolls and Cotton Pellets

Use

Cotton rolls are used in all procedures:
- To dry an area
- For isolation
- To provide a rest for the evacuation tip
- To apply topical anesthetic
- To retract tissues

Cotton pellets are used to:
- Dry tissues and tooth structures
- Place dental materials, such as cavity varnish

Parts

Cotton rolls are made of super absorbent and non-linting cotton. They are either smooth or braided with silky yarn. Cotton pellets are small balls of absorbent cotton. Both cotton rolls and cotton pellets come in several sizes.

Misc.

- Some cotton rolls are designed not to adhere to mucous membranes or sensitive tissues.
- Cotton rolls are available in different lengths and widths, both sterile and nonsterile, and roll dispensers are available.
- Cotton pellets come in different sizes, and containers designed for easy dispensing are available.

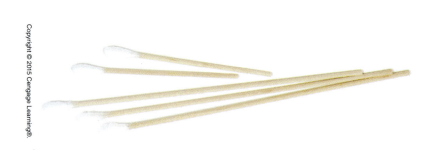

Cotton-Tipped Applicators

Use	• To dry and remove debris from the oral cavity and the tooth
	• To apply dental materials
	• To apply topical anesthetic

| **Parts** | Wood handles with tightly wrapped cotton tips |

Misc.	• Available in 3-inch and 6-inch lengths
	• Some are sealed in autoclavable bags of 100 tips.
	• Disposable

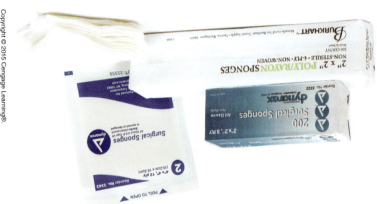

Gauze Sponges

Use

Gauze sponges have many functions, including their use in:
- Moisture absorption
- Retraction of tissues such as the tongue, cheeks, and lips
- Receiving debris or teeth/tooth fragments
- Keeping instruments clean during a procedure
- Application of pressure to bleeding area
- Disinfecting equipment, instruments, and the procedure area

Parts

Gauze sponges are folded pure virgin white cotton gauze; some are filled with 100 percent cotton fiber filling.

Misc.

- Gauze sponges are available in various sizes (e.g., 2 × 2, 3 × 3, 4 × 4, and 5 × 5), and they come filled and unfilled.
- Nonwoven sponges, which are made of a rayon/polyester blend, are also available. These sponges are softer, very absorbent, and are less adhesive to the wound. The unfilled sponges come in 4, 8, and 12 ply (layers).
- Both sterile and nonsterile gauze sponges are available. They are usually purchased by the case but also can be purchased in individual presterilized packets of two cotton-filled sponges.

Face Masks and Shields Used in Dentistry

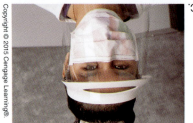

C.

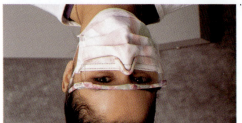

B.

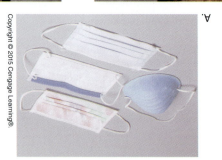

A.

Use

Face masks and shields are part of infection control techniques to prevent the spread of disease by protecting the dentist and dental auxiliary from exposure to blood, debris, and dust while performing skills/tasks. Masks and shields prevent cross-contamination between the dental team members and the patient.

Parts

One-piece masks are made of soft white facial tissue. There are inner and outer layers designed to resist moisture and to prevent irritation for sensitive skin. These masks are secured in place with elastic loops that fit around the ears or with ties that tie in the back of the head. Other masks are molded and are constructed of several layers of fluid-resistant material. Most masks have a flexible aluminum nosepiece that secures the mask around the nose to prevent safety glasses from fogging.

Shields are clear, distortion free, and fog free, and wrap around the face for protection. They are held in place by a soft or hard plastic headband.

A. Face masks in a variety of types, colors, and designs
B. Face mask in place with eyewear
C. Face mask in place with shield

Misc.

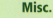

- Face masks should be worn with shields or eyewear.
- Face masks are disposable.
- Face shields can be disinfected and replaced when needed.

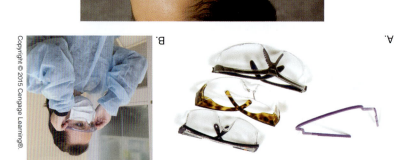

C.

B.

A.

Protective Eyewear

Use

Protective eyewear protects the eyes of the dentist, assistant, and patient from blood, saliva, and debris during dental treatment. Eyewear also offers protection from infectious diseases and aerosol droplets that may be transferred during treatment.

Parts

Eye protection used in dentistry consists of eyeglass frames and lenses, which are usually made of lightweight plastic material.

A. Example of protective eyewear
B. Eyewear on dental assistant

Misc.

- Eyewear comes in many styles and colors, and is often adjustable. All styles are designed to provide eye protection from the side, front, and top.
- Anti-fog products are available to minimize fogging. Eyewear can be run under warm water to reduce fogging.
- If glasses are worn, side shields (Figure C) or goggles can be worn over them to ensure protection.
- The lenses of some eyewear are amber, grey, or dark; such eyewear is worn when the curing light is used during a procedure.
- Preassembled disposable eye shields are available.
- Eyewear needs to fit properly and be comfortable so that it can be worn for long periods of time.

A.

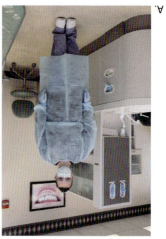

B.

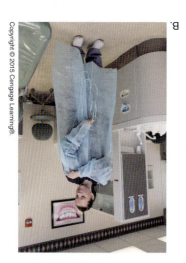

Use

Gowns are used to cover clothing and protect from saliva, blood, debris, and fluids during dental treatment and sterilization procedures.

Parts

Disposable gowns are made with polyethylene or polypropylene; have long sleeves, often with elastic or knit cuffs; and are constructed to fit closely around the neck. The length can be jacket length, at the knee, or longer.

A. Example of disposable protective gown that is knee length
B. Example of a dental assistant placing a protective gown

Misc.

- Gowns should be impervious to most liquids and aerosols.
- Gowns can be disposable or made from fabric for continued use.
- Both types are available in many colors and styles.
- Gowns should be changed daily or when contamination occurs.
- Gowns should be removed prior to leaving the dental office.

C.

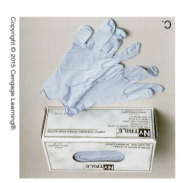

B.

A.

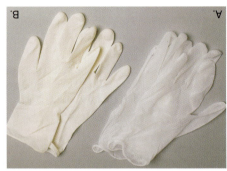

Examination Gloves

Use

Gloves are used as a barrier to microorganisms. Gloves are worn to protect the dental team members from contact with saliva, blood, and debris.

Parts

Examination gloves are made of several types of materials, including latex, nitrile, and vinyl. Gloves fit either the right or left hand and may be powdered or powder free. They come in a variety of sizes, from extra-small through extra-large.

A. Vinyl gloves
B. Latex examination gloves
C. Lightly powdered, colored nitrile examination gloves

Misc.

- Some gloves are scented, and some offer more tactile sensitivity and a nonslip grip on the fingertips.
- Nitrile and vinyl gloves are designed for dental assistants and patients with latex sensitivity.
- Gloves are available in nonsterile (worn for most dental treatment) and sterile (for surgical treatment) types.
- Gloves are worn over the cuffs of the protective gown.
- Gloves are purchased in boxes of 100.
- If gloves are penetrated or torn, or if the user leaves the area, the gloves should be removed, hands washed, and new gloves placed before treatment continues.

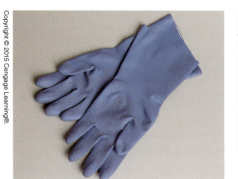

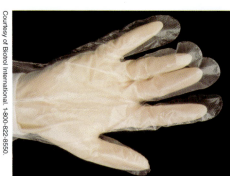

Overgloves and Utility Gloves

| **Use** | Overgloves are used to prevent cross-contamination. They are worn over examination gloves or alone when something outside the treatment area needs to be handled. An example would be holding a patient chart or if the assistant needs to retrieve an instrument from another area. |

Utility gloves are used when disinfecting the dental unit and in the sterilizing area when cleaning and preparing instruments and trays. They are used for protection when handling hazardous materials.

Parts Overgloves are clear polyethylene gloves that are sometimes textured. They are nonpowdered and nonsterile.

Utility gloves come in a variety of colors and sizes to fit the left and right hands. They are one-piece, heavy-duty vinyl/nitrile gloves.

Misc.
- Overgloves come in a box or bag of 100 or more. They are often referred to as food-handler gloves. They are available in numerous sizes.
- The fingers of utility gloves are textured to prevent slippage. They are puncture and chemical resistant. Each individual should have his or her own gloves. They should be washed thoroughly after each use.

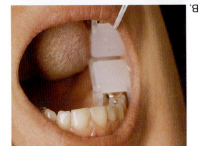

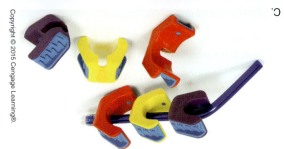

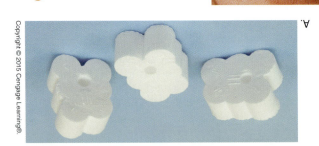

Mouth Props

Use

Props are used to assist the patient in keeping his or her mouth open during treatment.

Parts

Mouth props are one-piece, wedge-shaped structures designed to fit the oral cavity. They may be made of rubber, plastic, or Styrofoam.

A. Styrofoam disposable mouth prop
B. Mouth prop in patient's mouth with ligature attached
C. Variety of sizes and colors of mouth props

Misc.

- Mouth props are placed in the posterior between the maxillary and mandibular teeth.
- They are available as disposable or autoclavable items.
- The come in a variety of colors and sizes from pediatric to adult.
- They are used often for sedated patients.
- For patient safety and to prevent choking, a ligature should be tied to the mouth prop.

B.

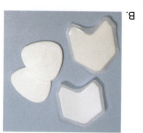

A.

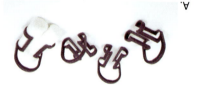

B.

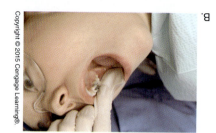

A.

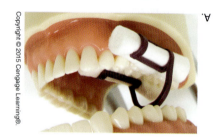

Use

Cotton roll holders are used to hold cotton rolls on buccal and lingual surfaces of the teeth in a specific area on the mandibular arch. They are also used to isolate, retract, and hold cotton rolls to keep an area dry.

Dry angles/dry aids are used to keep the mouth dry by covering the Stensen's (parotid) duct to restrict the flow of saliva. They absorb saliva and keep the working area dry. They also protect the cheek during dental treatment.

The backing on dry angles reflects light to improve visibility.

Parts

A. A cotton roll holder is a one-piece plastic device with two clamps sized to hold a cotton roll connected with a flexible bow.

B. Dry angles/dry aids are thin absorbent wafers/pads. They are angular in shape, with one side made of absorbent cotton and the other side consisting of moisture-proof backing. Some have a silver backing that reflects light into the oral cavity.

Misc.

- Cotton roll holders may be disposable or Garmer clamps made of stainless steel that can be sterilized. They are available in different sizes and colors.
- Dry angles restrict the flow of saliva from the parotid gland for up to 15 minutes. They are considered a cotton roll substitute.
- Dry angles are ideal for bonding procedures, sealant application, placement of restorations, and cementation.

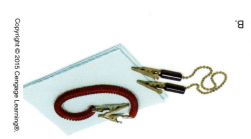

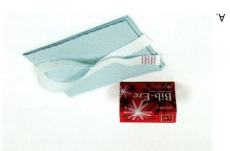

B.

A.

Patient Bibs and Bib Holders

| **Use** | Bibs cover the patient for protection from moisture and debris. Bib clips hold the bib in place. |
| **Parts** | Patient bibs are two- or three-ply tissue with poly backing. Bib holders have two clips connected by a tube, strip, and chain or coiled expandable plastic. |

A. Patient disposable bibs and disposable bib holders
B. Disposable bib with bib clips

Misc.
- Patient bibs come in a variety of sizes and contours, and are disposable.
- They may be purchased in many colors and printed designs with different features.
- Some bids come with adhesive tabs so that bib clips are not required to secure the bib on the patient.
- Bib clips can be disposable, disinfected, and/or autoclavable.

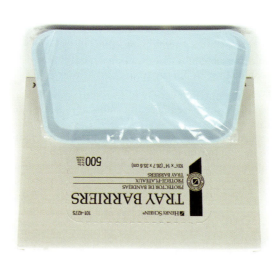

Tray Covers

Use Tray covers are used to cover the trays that are used to hold dental instruments, supplies, and materials used for a specific procedure; they protect the tray from moisture/liquid that may occur during a procedure.

Parts Made from heavyweight paper or a polyethylene-backed paper

Misc.
- Tray covers come in many sizes to cover all sizes of trays.
- Tray covers come in many colors and several designs.
- Some offices use tray covers on the counter or cart without a tray.
- Tray covers impede the flow of moisture and protect the surface.

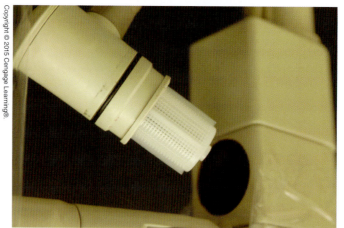

Traps, Screens, and Filters

Use	• Traps, screens, and filters are used to catch debris from the salvia ejector and high-volume evacuation (HVE) systems.
	• They keep evacuation systems from becoming clogged with debris and reducing the efficiency during a procedure.
Parts	• Traps, screens, and filters are usually one-piece plastic devices designed to adapt to the different types of dental equipment.
	• They are ordered by unit type and system utilized.
	• The image here shows a high-volume disposable trap shown on the unit.
Misc.	• Traps, screens, and filters come in many shapes, sizes, and designs.
	• These traps, screens, and filters are disposable.

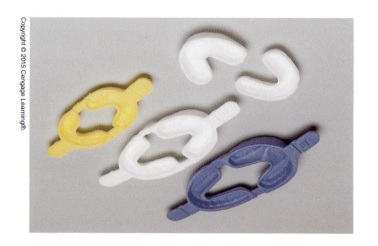

Fluoride Trays

Use	They are used to hold the fluoride gel/solution in the mouth around the teeth.
Parts	Dual-arch trays, fold-over trays, or single-arch applicator trays normally made from closed-cell foam
Misc.	<ul><li>Available in multiple colors and sizes</li><li>Disposable</li><li>Available in single-arch, double-fold-over, and dual-arch trays with a saliva ejector feature</li><li>Some folding-design trays have locking handles that allow for easy placement and removal.</li><li>They are often sold in amounts of 50 or 100.</li></ul>

Surface Barriers

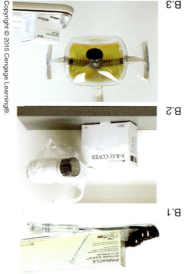

B.3

B.2

B.1

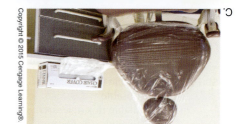

C.

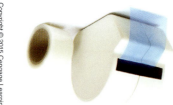

A.

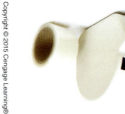

| **Use** | Improve infection control, prevent cross-contamination, protect surfaces, give the patient confidence in the infection control techniques used by the dentist |
| **Parts** | **A.** Perforated control film with adhesive backing |

Use

Improve infection control, prevent cross-contamination, protect surfaces, give the patient confidence in the infection control techniques used by the dentist

Parts

A. Perforated control film with adhesive backing
- Comes in 4 × 6″ and 2 1/2 × 6″
- Available in colors, clear, or designed
- Most often used with dispenser

B. Sleeves/sheaths: Medical-grade plastic that is available in many sizes and shapes to cover most equipment in dental treatment rooms
  - B.1 Syringe sleeve
  - B.2 X-ray cover
  - B.3 Covers for light handles

C. Chair cover: Medical-grade plastic that is available in half- and full-chair cover designed to fit the variety of dental chairs

Misc.

- These barriers are disposable and are designed for easy placement and removal.
- There are barriers to cover everything in the dental treatment room, from the dental chair to the handpieces, dental light, curing light, impression gun, air-water syringe, high-volume evacuator (HVE) handle and saliva ejector, computer keyboards, sensor covers, x-ray tubeheads and controls, and instruments and trays.
- Surface barriers are designed to be easy to place and remove for efficient room turn-around.

E.

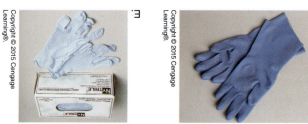

D.

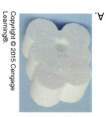

C.

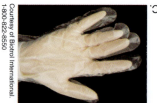

B.

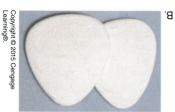

A.

_____ 1. Which item is used to control saliva?

_____ 2. Which item is used to prop the mouth open?

_____ 3. Which type of glove is used while disinfecting the dental unit?

_____ 4. Which type of glove is often called the food-handler's glove?

_____ 5. Which type of glove is used for patient treatment?

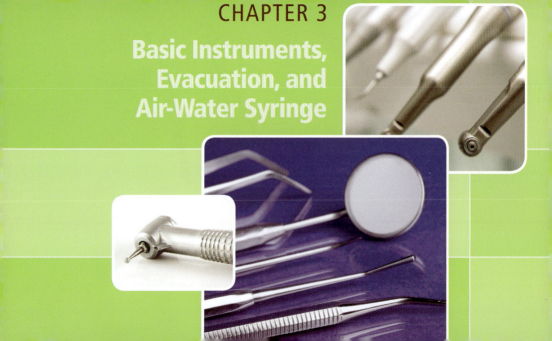

CHAPTER 3

Basic Instruments, Evacuation, and Air-Water Syringe

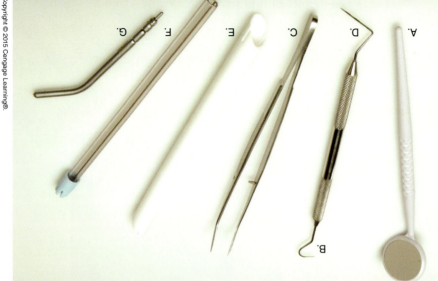

Basic Examination Instruments

Use

The basic tray setup includes instruments that are used for the examination of the oral cavity and the dentition. They can be used alone for the initial examination and are found on procedure tray setups. The primary instruments on the basic tray setup are the mouth mirror, explorer, cotton pliers, and periodontal probe. These instruments are used with the evacuator, saliva ejector, and air-water syringe.

Parts

The basic tray setup includes:
A. Mouth mirror
B. Explorer
C. Cotton pliers/forceps
D. Periodontal probe
E. Evacuator tip
F. Saliva ejector
G. Three-way syringe tip (also called air-water syringe tip)

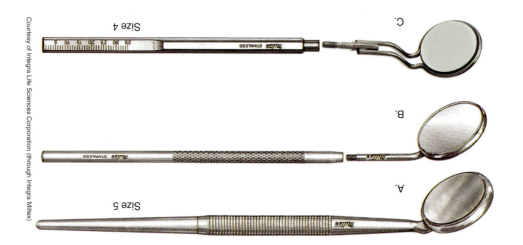

Mouth Mirror

A.

B.

C.

Size 5

Size 4

STAINLESS

STAINLESS

35 30 25 20 15 10 5

Use	• To provide indirect vision in the oral cavity
	• To reflect light into the mouth to illuminate an area being examined
	• To retract oral tissues such as the lips, tongue, and cheeks
	• To reflect light (transillumination) through the tooth surface to detect fractures
	• To protect tissues from the handpiece or bur
Parts	**A.** Single-ended instrument made of plastic or metal
	B and C. Straight handle with option of removable replacement head
Misc.	• Mirrors are available in different sizes and types.
	• Common sizes of mirrors are #4 and #5.
	• Front-surface mirrors are more accurate and give a clear view.
	• Concave-surface mirrors magnify the image.
	• Flat-surface mirrors are used in the disposable models.
	• Plane- or regular-surface mirrors reflect from the back of the glass and give a "ghost-like" image.

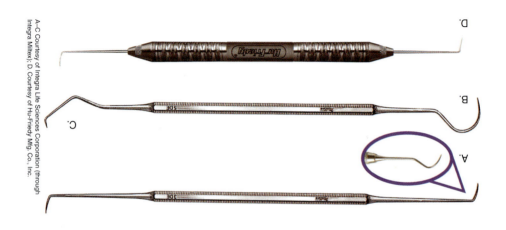

Explorer

A–C Courtesy of Integra Life Sciences Corporation (through Integra Miltex); D. Courtesy of Hu-Friedy Mfg. Co., Inc.

D.

B.

C.

A.

Use	• To examine the tooth structure for any defects or areas of decay
	• To examine restorations and check for faulty margins or fractures
	• To remove excess materials from around the margins of restorations or from bases and liners in the cavity preparation
Parts	**A.** Pigtail
	B. Shepherd's hook
	C. Orban, also called #17
	D. Right angle
Misc.	• Explorers can be single or double ended.
	• The end is characterized by a thin, sharp point of flexible steel.
	• Explorers come in a variety of angles and with several different ends.

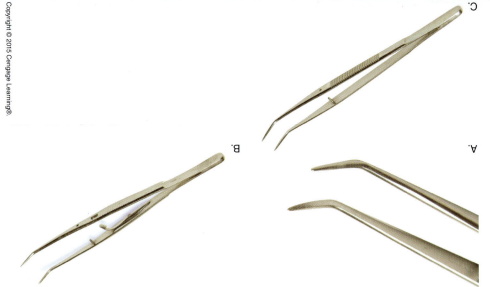

Cotton Forceps (Pliers)

A.

B.

C.

Use	To place and remove items from the oral cavity, such as cotton rolls, cotton pellets, wedges, and large pieces of debris
Parts	**A.** Ends can be smooth or serrated on the beaks.
	B. Handles can be locking.
	C. Handles can be non-locking.
Misc.	• Cotton forceps (pliers) are shaped like large tweezers.
	• The ends can be smooth or serrated (A) on the beaks.
	• May have either locking (B) or non-locking handles (C).
	• The tips may be angled or straight.

A.

B.

Courtesy of Integra Life Sciences Corporation (through Integra Miltex)

Expro

- The expro is a combination instrument that has an explorer on one end and a periodontal probe on the other end.
- Cuts down on the number of instruments needed on the tray

Parts

A. Explorer end
B. Periodontal probe end

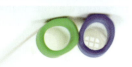

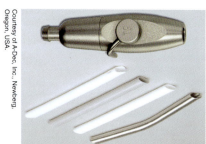

Use	• To remove fluids and debris from the oral cavity

Use
- To remove fluids and debris from the oral cavity
- To retract soft tissues
- To prevent discomfort to soft tissue
- Screens prevent crowns, inlays, veneers, excess materials, etc. from being lost into the evacuation system.

Parts
- Evacuator tips
- Evacuator handle
- Plastic sleeve with a beveled screen that sits over the end of the evacuator tip

Misc.
- Placed into the evacuator handle that is connected to the high-volume evacuation system
- Made from metal or plastic
- Tips can be rubber coated for patient comfort
- Straight or curved
- Tips normally beveled
- The screens can be used on all standard plastic and metal evacuator tips.
- Low cost
- Screens are purchased in bags of 100.

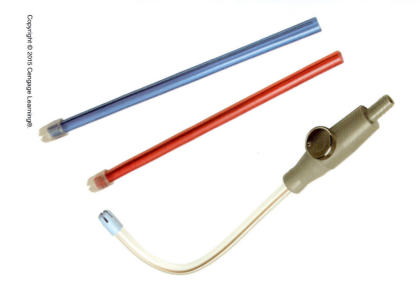

Saliva Ejector

Use	• A low-volume (low-velocity) evacuation system used to remove fluids from the oral cavity
Parts	• Flexible, plastic tube about one-third in diameter of the size of the high-volume evacuation tip • Bendable with a guard cover on the end that is placed into the patient's mouth
Misc.	• Disposable • Available in multiple colors • Used primarily on mandibular arch • Commonly used during coronal polish, sealant, and fluoride procedures • Used during preventative treatment when the operator does not have an assistant • Some are designed with a soft smooth tip to prevent patient discomfort.

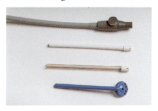 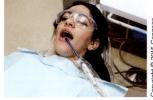

Copyright © 2015 Cengage Learning®.

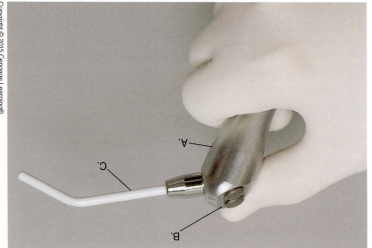

A.

B.

C.

Three-Way Syringe Tip/Air-Water Syringe Tip

Use
- Emits water, air, or a combination of both in a spray
- Directs the air, water, or spray
- Used for retraction of the tongue, cheeks, lips, and tissues of the oral cavity

Parts
A. Handle
B. Controls
C. Disposable tip

Misc.
- Allows water or air or spray to dispense
- Plastic or metal
- Disposable or able to be sterilized

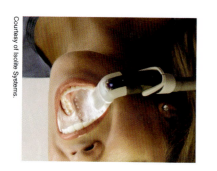

Courtesy of Isolite Systems.

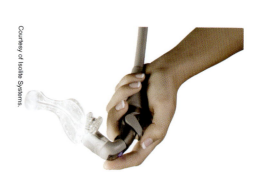

Courtesy of Isolite Systems.

Isolite System

Use	• Provides isolation, retraction, evacuation, and a light source in one piece of equipment. It also provides a mouth prop for the patient.
Parts	• Titanium control head, power/vacuum hose, and a one-time-use mouthpiece • The control head contains a light emitter, a dual-channel vacuum, and controls for both. • The system is connected to the dental unit vacuum system and an electrical source.
Misc.	• The mouthpiece is available in different sizes. • The mouthpiece is disposable. • The light setting can be controlled for light-sensitive material. • The mouthpiece isolates an entire quadrant and can be used on both the maxillary and mandibular arches.

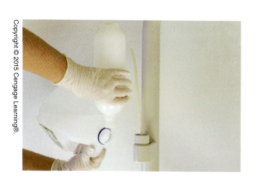
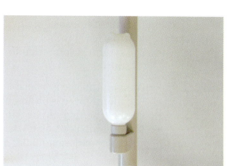

Self-Contained Water Unit and Water Line Treatments

Use	• A reservoir that houses quality water to be used by dental handpieces and air-water syringe. It aids in the control and prevention of water contamination.
	• Evacuation system cleaners are used after each patient, at the end of the day, and at the end of the week to keep the evacuation system clean and odor free, and to prevent buildup of debris from blood, salvia, tissue, and dental materials such as fluoride inside the lines.
Parts	• Plastic bottles that attach to the dental unit
	• Designed with a cap and a plastic tube where the plastic bottle attaches
	• Evacuation system cleaners can be tablets, solutions, packets, or systems that are usually mixed and then suctioned into the tubing. Some systems require the solution to sit for a few minutes, and others require repeated flushing.
Misc.	• The water is filled when empty and tablets can be added prior to each filling to prevent odor and foul taste due to bacteria.
	• The system is cleaned following the manufacturer's directions.
	• The Centers for Disease Control and Prevention (CDC) requests ongoing monitoring of water lines.
	• There are numerous evacuation cleaners that can be used to clean, deodorize, and decontaminate water lines.

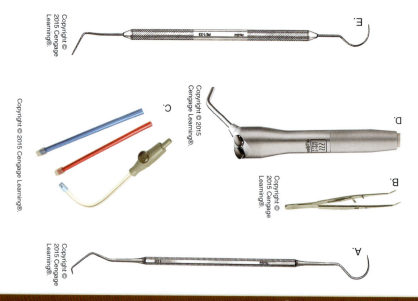

E.

D.

C.

B.

A.

_____ 1. Which instrument is used to transport items to and from the oral cavity?

_____ 2. Which instrument is called the expro?

_____ 3. Which instrument is called the explorer?

_____ 4. Which instrument emits water, air, or a combination of both in a spray?

_____ 5. Which instrument is called a saliva ejector?

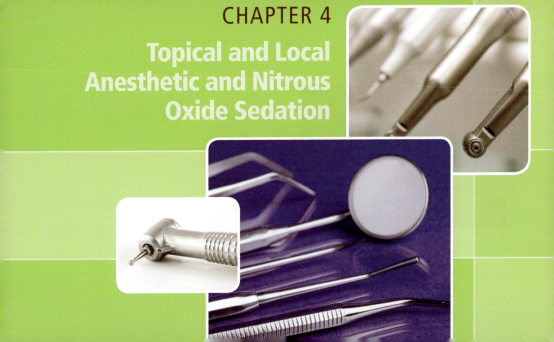

CHAPTER 4

Topical and Local Anesthetic and Nitrous Oxide Sedation

A.

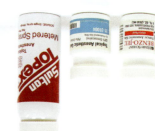

B.

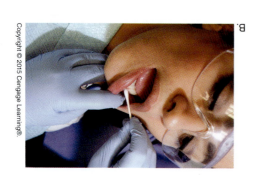

Use	Topical anesthetics are placed on the surface of the oral mucosa to desensitize the tissue for a brief period of time. They are used prior to placement of local anesthetic, during subgingival scaling, during root planing, when seating crowns, in dental dam placement, when placing matrix bands, when taking radiographs, for suppressing the gag reflex, and sometimes for periodontal probing. Topical anesthetic comes in gels, ointments, liquids, metered sprays, patches and single doses.
Parts	**A.** Ointments and metered spray **B.** Placing topical anesthetic on a patient
Misc.	Most topical anesthetics are flavored.

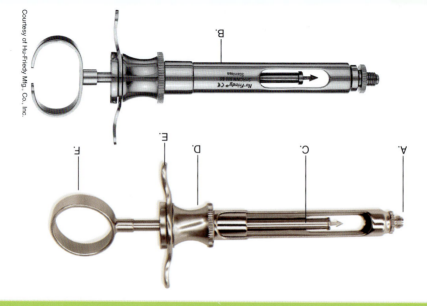

Courtesy of Hu-Friedy Mfg. Co., Inc.

| **Use** | • To administer local anesthetic to a specific area. The American Dental Association (ADA) recommends the aspirating syringe. |
| | • The harpoon is securely placed in the rubber stopper, which then allows the operator to check the position of the needle. |

Parts

A. Threaded end (needle adapter)
B. Syringe barrel
C. Piston rod with harpoon
D. Finger grip
E. Finger bar
F. Thumb ring

Misc.

• Local anesthetic syringes are autoclavable.
• An anesthetic syringe without a harpoon is known as a non-aspirating syringe.
• Many anesthetic syringes must have the piston rod with harpoon retracted to allow insertion of the cartridge.

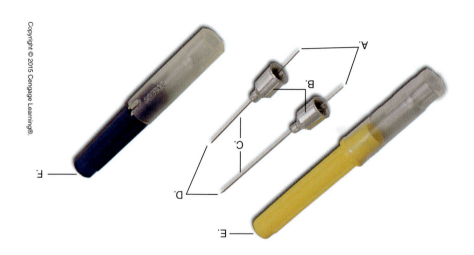

A.

B.

C.

D.

E.

F.

Local Anesthetic Needle

| **Use** | • To penetrate the tissues |
| | • To direct the local anesthetic solution from the carpule (anesthetic cartridge) into the surrounding tissues |

Parts

A. Syringe end
B. Hub
C. Shank
D. Bevel
E. Long needle: used for administration of nerve block injections
F. Short needle: used for administration of infiltration and field block injections

Misc.

• Needles come in different gauges or diameters. The most common are 25, 27, and 40 gauges.
• With anesthetic needles, the smaller the gauge of the needle, the larger the diameter of the needle.

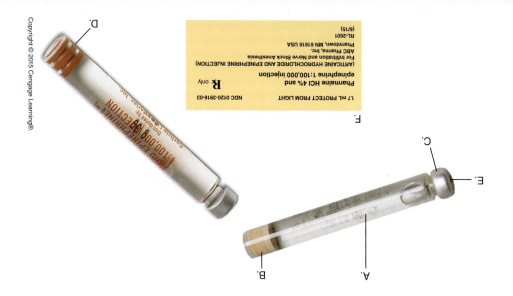

Local Anesthetic Cartridge

A.

B.

C.

D.

E.

F.

NDC 0120-3916-03

R only

Pharmaine HCl 4% and
epinephrine 1:100,000 Injection

(ARTICAINE HYDROCHLORIDE AND EPINEPHRINE INJECTION)
For Infiltration and Nerve Block Anesthesia

ABC Pharma, Inc.
Pharmtown, MN 61616 USA

RL-2601
(6/15)

1.7 mL PROTECT FROM LIGHT

| **Use** | The anesthetic cartridge, also called the carpule, is a glass cylinder that contains the anesthetic solution. |

Parts

A. Glass cartridge (carpule)
B. Rubber stopper or plunger: where the harpoon of syringe inserts
C. Aluminum cap
D. Color coding of local anesthetic (required by the ADA)
E. Diaphragm: where the needle inserts
F. Mylar plastic label: prevents breakage and provides identification information, including type of anesthetic, percentage of anesthetic, with or without epinephrine, strength of epinephrine, and expiration date.

Misc.

- Local anesthetics follow the ADA color-coding band, which indicates types of anesthetic and vasoconstrictor combinations.
- Cartridges should be carefully examined for expired shelf-life date, large bubbles, extruded plungers, corrosion, or rust. All of these are reasons for cartridges to be discarded.
- The rubber stopper or plunger is slightly indented.
- The higher percentage of epinephrine (vasoconstrictor), the longer the anesthetic lasts.

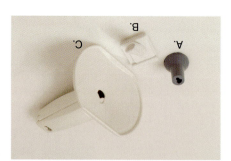

A.

B.

C.

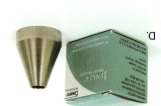

D.

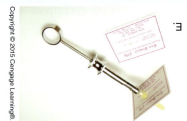

E.

Recapping Devices and Needle Stick Protection

Use
- Recapping devices are used to hold the needle cap; this allows the operator to safely recap the needle after delivery of anesthetic. The recapping devices help to prevent needlesticks.
- Needlestick guards prevent needle stick injury when capping and recapping the needle. They protect the dental assistant, dentist, and dental hygienist when recapping the needle.

Parts
- **A.** Rubber recapping device
- **B.** Needle capper
- **C.** Handheld recapping device
- **D.** The Jenker Needlestick protector
- **E.** The needle stick guard is a square of cardboard material with a hole in the middle for the needle cap. Needle guard shown on needle cap and syringe.

Misc.
- The needle is slid into the protective guard using one hand or by placing the needle of the syringe in a mechanical recapping device.
- Most recapping devices can be sterilized.
- The needlestick guard is placed after the needle is placed on the syringe.
- The needle can be capped and recapped with one hand when using the needle guard.
- At no time should fingers or the thumb be in the front toward the syringe of the needle guard.
- The needle guard also acts as a prop to hold the syringe when it is not in use
- Needle guards are available in boxes/packs of 100 or 500

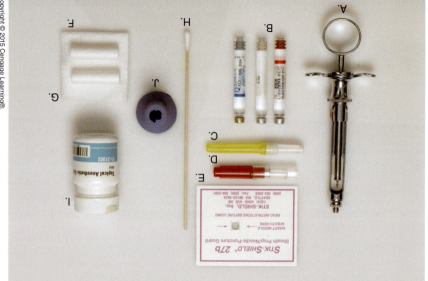

Use

Instruments and materials needed to place topical and local anesthetic are assembled on the treatment tray. Usually the anesthetic tray setup is part of the procedure tray.

Parts

A. Aspirating syringe
B. Selection of local anesthetic cartridges
C. Long needle
D. Short needle
E. Needlestick shield
F. Cotton rolls
G. 2 × 2 gauze sponge
H. Cotton-tip applicator
I. Topical anesthetic
J. Recapping device

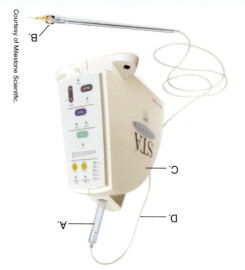

Courtesy of Milestone Scientific.

Local Anesthetic—Computer-Controlled Delivery System (The Wand)

| **Use** | This is a system to administer single-tooth, palatal, mandibular, and all other injections. The system's microprocessor delivers a controlled pressure and volume of anesthetic solution at a rate that is below the pain threshold. |

Parts

A. Standard anesthetic cartridge
B. Any size or gauge of anesthetic needle
C. Microprocessing unit
D. Plastic microtubing
E. Foot control (not pictured)

Misc.

- It is used with a pen-like grasp that allows for flexibility in administration.
- The auxiliary can prepare the Wand/STA prior to treatment, similar to the anesthetic syringe.
- The computer manages the flow of the anesthetic while the operator focuses on needle placement.
- It improves ergonomics for the operator while increasing patient comfort.

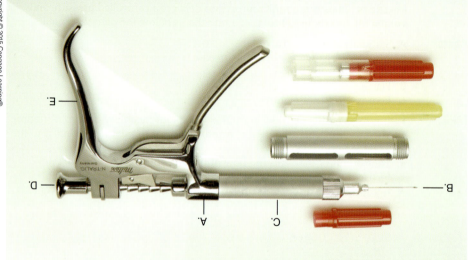

Local Anesthetic—Periodontal Ligament Injection Syringe

Use	Delivers a precise amount of anesthesia to one or two teeth in a quadrant and is sometimes used as an adjunct to another injection where the patient is only partially anesthetized
Parts	**A.** Pressure syringe **B.** Needle end **C.** Barrel **D.** Plunger **E.** Handle

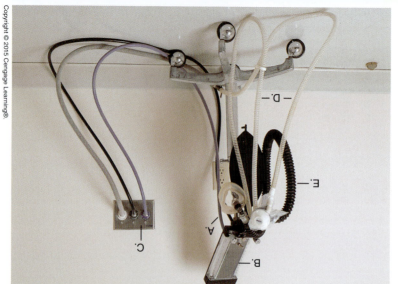

Nitrous Oxide Sedation Equipment

Use	• To provide relaxation
	• To relieve apprehension for patients during dental treatment
Parts	**A.** Nitrous oxide and oxygen gases are used together to allow a safe method of sedation.
	B. The nitrous oxide unit has controls and gauges to administer the proper amount of nitrous and oxygen.
	C. Hoses connect to a tank of nitrous oxide and a tank of oxygen.
	D. Breathing tubes (hoses) connect the nitrous oxide and oxygen tanks to the nasal hoods for administration.
	E. Each unit has a scavenger system to carry away exhaled and additional gas.

A.

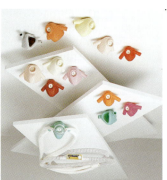

B.

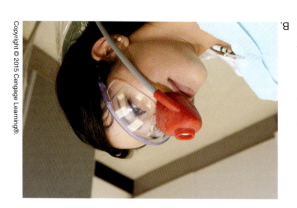

Use	Placed over the patient's nose so that the gases flow through to the patient
Parts	

- Rubber nose covers that come in a variety of colors
- They are attached to a scavenging circuit.
- Some are scented for patient comfort.
- Attach to the breathing tubes that come from the nitrous oxide tank and the oxygen tank

A. Variety of color-coded nasal hoods/nosepieces

B. Patient with nasal hood/nosepiece in place

Test Your Knowledge

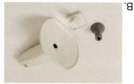

B.

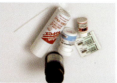

E.

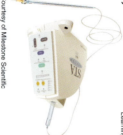

Courtesy of Milestone Scientific

C.

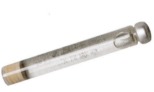

A.

D.

_____ 1. These devices are used to place the needle cap back on after the anesthetic has been given to the patient.

_____ 2. This system is used to deliver a precise amount of anesthesia to one or two teeth in a quadrant.

_____ 3. This is a glass cylinder that contains the anesthetic solution.

_____ 4. This is a method of anesthetic delivery in which a computer controls the amount of anesthetic administered.

_____ 5. This material numbs the tissue before the anesthetic needle is placed.

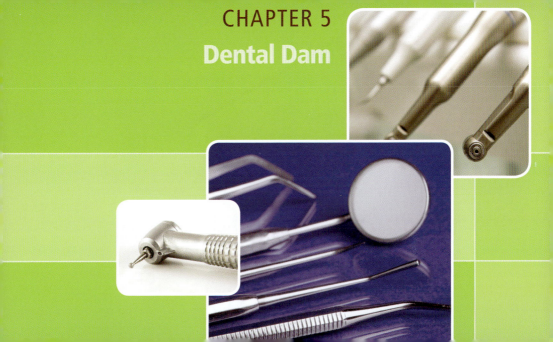

CHAPTER 5
Dental Dam

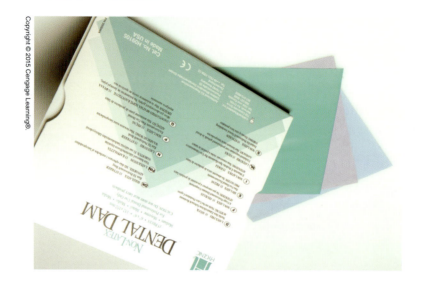

Dental Dam

| **Use** | • To isolate teeth for dental procedures |
| | • To keep the area clean and dry while performing dental procedures |

Use

- To isolate teeth for dental procedures
- To keep the area clean and dry while performing dental procedures

Parts

- Made from either latex or latex-free material
- Comes in sizes 4 × 4 inches, 5 × 5 inches, 6 × 6 inches, or a continuous roll

Misc.

- The dental dam is often referred to as the rubber dam.
- Available in a wide range of colors, including green, blue, and pastels
- Colors allow for increased visibility and contrast.
- Scented and flavored dams also are available.
- Available in a variety of thicknesses: thin (light), medium, and heavy

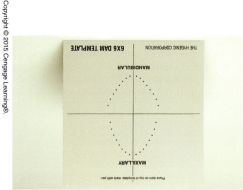

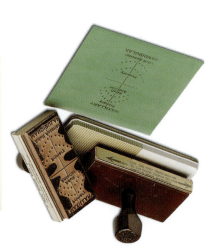

Dental Dam Stamp and Template

Use
- The stamp is used to mark where the holes should be punched for correct dental dam placement.
- The template is used as a guide for marking the correct position for punching holes for dental dam placement.

Parts
- The stamp has 32 dots located on a punch and is used with a stamp pad to mark the rubber dam material.
- The template is made of durable plastic and has holes where an ink pen can be used to mark the correct position for punching.

Misc.
- The operator should examine the oral cavity before punching the dental dam to adjust positioning for the specific patient's dentition.

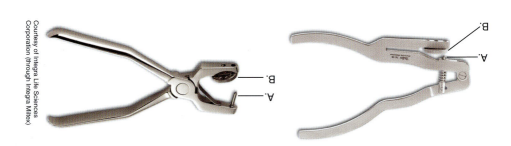

Courtesy of Integra Life Sciences
Corporation (through Integra Miltex)

A.

B.

A.

B.

Dental Dam Punch

Use	To punch holes in dental dam for each identified tooth the dentist wants isolated
Parts	**A.** A stylus, which is a sharp projection to punch through the dental dam
	B. A punch table or plate, which is a rotating disc containing several hole sizes
	• No. 1 hole size (smallest hole)–Used for lower incisors
	• No. 2 hole size–Used for upper incisors
	• No. 3 hole size–Used for premolars and cuspids
	• No. 4 hole size–Used for molars
	• No. 5 hole size (largest hole)–Used for molars and the anchor tooth
Misc.	• The operator should examine the oral cavity before punching the dental dam to adjust positioning for the specific patient's dentition.
	• The space between the holes is approximately 3 to 3.5 mm.

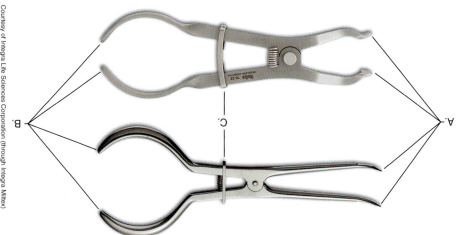

Dental Dam Forceps

A.

B.

C.

To place and remove the dental dam clamp

A. Two beaks that fit into the holes of the jaws of the clamp

B. Handle (where the pressure is applied to open the beaks)

C. Lock (sliding bar) that keeps the beaks of the forceps open to secure the clamp in position until it is placed on the anchor tooth. The sliding bar can be released once the clamp is placed, and then the beaks of the forceps will come together.

Misc.

- The forceps open with a spring motion.

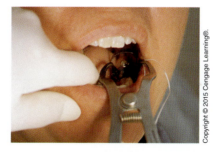

Copyright © 2015 Cengage Learning®.

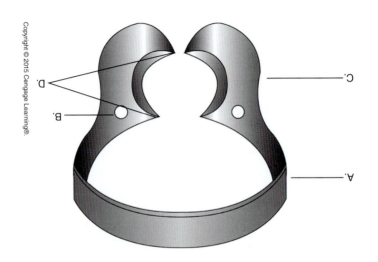

Dental Dam Clamp

A.

B.

C.

D.

Use	To stabilize and secure the dental dam material in place
Parts	**A.** Bow (connects the jaws of the clamps and is positioned to the distal)
	B. Forceps hole (utilized by the forceps to place the clamp)
	C. Jaw (rounded part of the clamp that fits tightly to the lingual and buccal/facial surfaces of the tooth)
	D. Jaw points (four points on the jaws of the clamp that are located at different widths and angles that fit to secure the clamp on the tooth near the cementoenamel junction)

Misc.

- The tooth to be clamped must be evaluated before the clamp selection is made.
- The width of the tooth must be about the same as the width medial/distal between the points of the jaws of the clamp.
- Ensure that the clamp fits tightly.
- Ligatures of dental floss should be tied to the bow as a safe measure in case the clamp dislodges from the tooth.
- Clamps that have the letter A following the number have jaws that bend sharply downward toward the gingival.
- Clamps without the letter A have jaws that are on a flat plane.

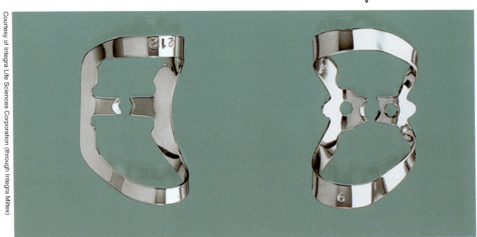

Anterior or Cervical Clamp

A.

Use	To stabilize and secure the dental dam material in place on an anterior tooth
Parts	Double bowed
	A. Two types of anterior clamps that are double bowed
	B. Anterior clamp in place on tooth number nine
Misc.	• Examples are the SSW 212 and the Hygienic B6 and B5.
	• Clamps are sterilized.
	• Dental floss ligatures are placed on clamps for rescue of a dislodged clamp.
	• Used for restorations and endodontic treatment on the anterior teeth

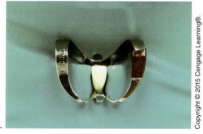

B.

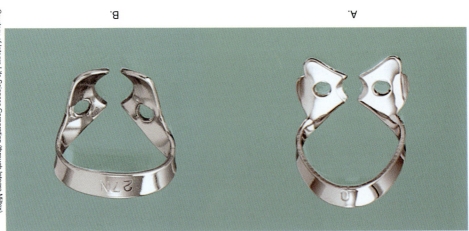

Premolar Clamp

Use   To stabilize and secure the dental dam material in place on a premolar

Parts   **A.** Winged
            B. Wingless

Misc.   - The clamp used is determined by tooth size and shape.
            - Dental floss ligatures are placed on clamps for rescue of a dislodged clamp.
            - Clamps are sterilized.
            - Variety of styles and sizes available

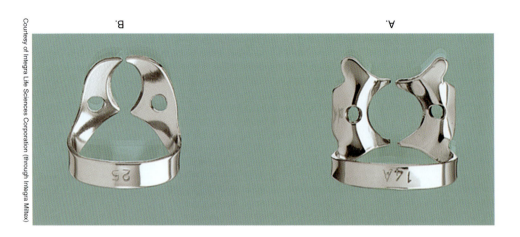

Universal Maxillary Clamp

A.

B.

Use

To stabilize and secure the dental dam material in place on a maxillary molar

Parts

A. Winged
B. Wingless

Misc.

- Can be used on right or left maxillary molars
- Variety of styles available
- Dental floss ligatures are placed on clamps for rescue of a dislodged clamp.
- Clamps are sterilized.
- Variety of sizes available

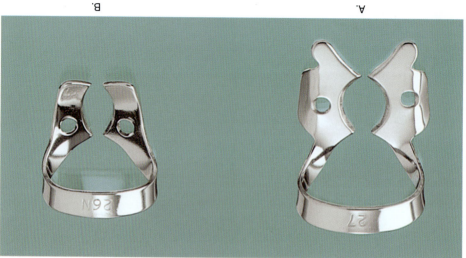

A.

B.

Universal Mandibular Clamp

Use	To stabilize and secure the dental dam material in place on a mandibular molar
Parts	**A.** Winged **B.** Wingless
Misc.	• Can be used on right or left mandibular molars • Variety of styles available • Dental floss ligatures are placed on clamps for rescue of a dislodged clamp. • Clamps are sterilized. • Variety of sizes available

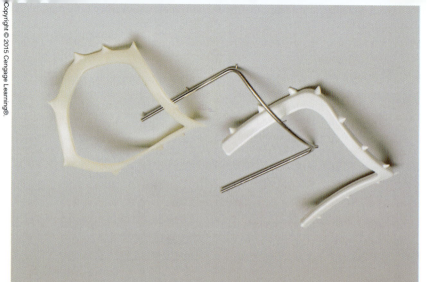

Dental Dam Frames

Use	Used to stretch and secure the dental dam in place across the patient's face
Parts	• U- or oval-shaped frames made from metal or plastic. • Small projections around the borders to secure the dental dam
Misc.	• Plastic frames are radiolucent. • The U-shaped frame is common and is known as the (metal) Young frame or (plastic) U-frame. • Frames can be placed over or under the dental dam material according to the dentist's preference. • Frames are sterilized. • The oval-shaped frame is known as the Ostby frame.

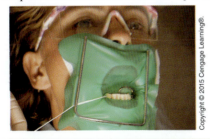

Copyright © 2015 Cengage Learning®.

A.

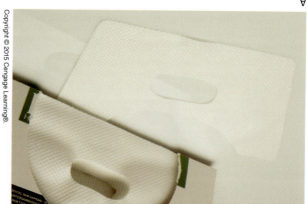

B.

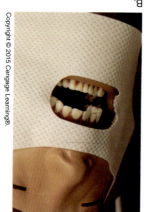

Use	For patient comfort and to absorb saliva, water, and perspiration

Parts
- **A.** Precut dental dam napkin
- **B.** Dental dam napkin with correct placement shown.
- Made of soft, absorbent fabric
- Precut
- Designed to prevent the dam material from touching the face by covering the area around the mouth and the cheeks

Misc.
- Available in several sizes
- Disposable

A.

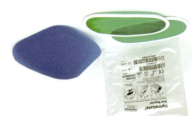

B.

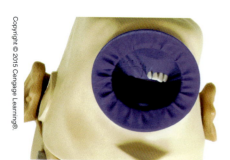

Use	For quick and easy placement of the dental dam for full-quadrant or single-use isolation
Parts	**A.** Latex pre-framed dental dams **B.** Dental dam placement
Misc.	• Available in several styles • Compact and comfortable for the patient • Easy placement for the operator • Disposable

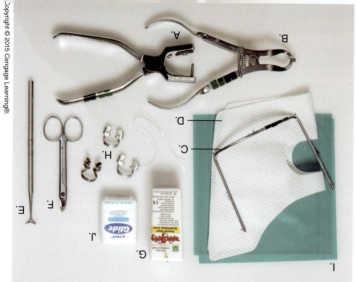

Dental Dam Tray Setup

Parts

A. Dental dam punch
B. Dental dam forceps
C. Dental dam frame
D. Dental dam napkin
E. Tucking instrument (T-ball burnisher)
F. Crown and bridge scissors
G. Widgets ligature (a stretchable cord placed like dental floss to hold the dental dam in place)
H. Clamps
I. Stamped dental dam
J. Dental floss (for inverting the dental dam material)

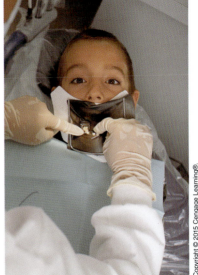

Copyright © 2015 Cengage Learning®.

A.

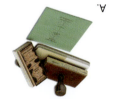

B.

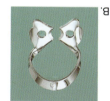

C.

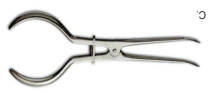

D.

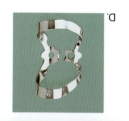

E.

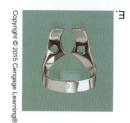

_____ 1. Which dental dam clamp is used for the anterior or cervical area?

_____ 2. Which dental dam clamp is used as a universal mandibular clamp?

_____ 3. Which dental dam clamp is used as a premolar clamp?

_____ 4. Which item is used to indicate where the dental dam should be punched?

_____ 5. Which item is the dental dam forceps?

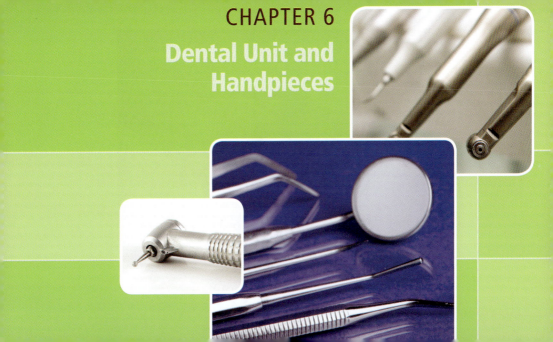

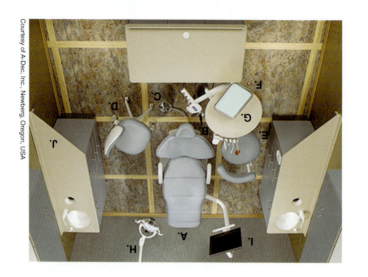

The Dental Delivery System

| **Use** | Comprehensive unit for delivering patient dental care |
| **Parts** | |

A. Ergonomically designed patient chair that provides comfort and support during treatment

B. Patient chair adjustments (not pictured)

C. Rheostat to control handpieces

D. Ergonomically designed chair for operator with lumbar support

E. Ergonomically designed chair for assistant with extended arm

F. Rear delivery system with air-water syringe, high-volume evacuator (HVE), and saliva ejector on assistant's side and handpieces and air-water syringe on operator's side.

G. Tray table for placement of tray setups and auxiliary items

H. Operating light attached to the dental unit or mounted on the ceiling

I. Computer screen for digital radiographs and patient information

J. Cabinetry with sinks and countertops

Misc.
- Units available in many sizes, designs, colors, and features to meet practice needs.
- The photo shown is of a rear delivery system; units are available with front and side delivery.
- Operator and assistant chairs need to be adjustable and have stable bases.
- Units are designed to allow for easy cleaning and disinfecting.

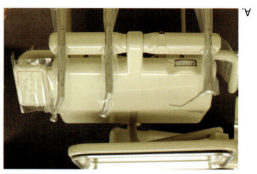

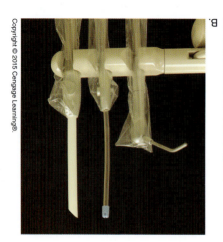

| **Use** | Provides placement of the air-water syringe, dental handpieces, HVE, saliva ejector, ultrasonic scaling unit, curing light, and other options used by the operator and the dental assistant. |

Parts
A. Unit shown with handpieces and air-water syringe used by the operator
B. Unit shown with air-water syringe, saliva ejector, and HVE used by the assistant

Misc.
- Units are plumbed with water and a vacuum system and electrical connections, including fiber optics.
- Units can be designed according to the operator's preference; for example, curing lights may be attached.
- Barriers are often placed over hard-to-clean areas.

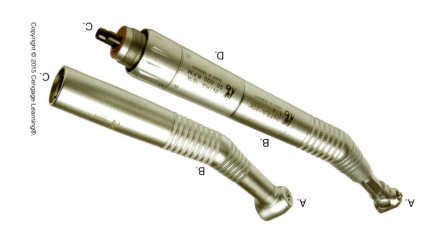

A.

B.

C.

D.

A.

B.

C.

The Parts of the Dental Handpiece

Use	Many dental handpieces are available for various procedures, both in the oral cavity and in the laboratory. Handpieces are used to remove dental decay, prepare the cavity preparation, polish the teeth, and polish and finish restorations and dental appliances.
Parts	**A.** Working end (head) where rotary instruments and attachments are held **B.** Shank-handle portion of the handpiece **C.** The connection end of the handpiece attaches to the power source here. **D.** Forward and reverse controls on the low-speed handpeice
Misc.	• Shown on the left is the low-speed handpiece with a prophy attachment; on the right is a high-speed handpiece. • All handpieces and attachments can be cleaned, lubricated, and sterilized; the manufacturer's directions should be followed.

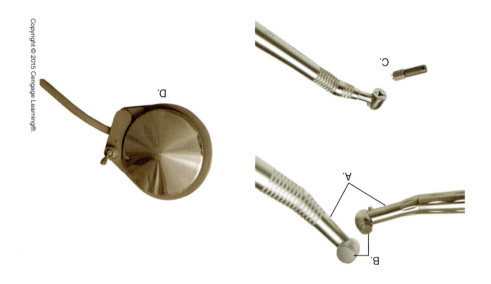

A.

B.

C.

D.

High-Speed Handpiece

| **Use** | The high-speed handpiece is used with a bur to rapidly cut teeth, as well as to smooth surfaces and finish restorations. |

Use

The high-speed handpiece is used with a bur to rapidly cut teeth, as well as to smooth surfaces and finish restorations.

Parts

A. High-speed handpiece
B. Button/release lever to allow for bur placement and removal
C. Chuck and bur tool to tighten and loosen the chuck
D. Rheostat (foot control of handpiece speed and water)

Misc.

- High-speed handpieces operate at 400,000 revolutions per minute (rpm) or higher.
- The high-speed handpiece produces frictional heat and must be cooled by a coolant such as air, water, or an air-water spray.
- The high-speed handpiece does not hold any attachments but does hold burs and other rotary instruments.
- The power source for the handpiece comes from compressed air. The rheostat is used to activate and control the speed of the handpiece. Also on the rheostat there is a switch to turn the water to the handpiece on or off.
- The burs are held in place by a small metal cylinder called a chuck. There are numerous ways to tighten or loosen the chuck; for example, either a bur tool/wrench or button/release lever on the back of the head of the handpiece may be used.

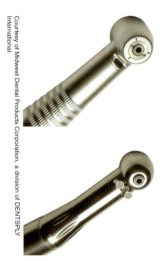

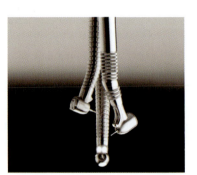

Fiber-Optic High-Speed Handpiece

Use

The fiber-optic system greatly improves the visibility of the treatment area by illuminating the area for the dentist.

Parts

Small illuminated area on the handpiece head that provides light during tooth preparation

Misc.

- The fiber-optic light is carried along optical bundles in the tubing of the handpiece.
- The light source for the fiber-optic light is placed in the head of the tubing where the fiber-optic handpiece attaches. This tubing attachment can only be used with the fiber-optic handpiece.
- Fiber-optic handpieces should only be attached to the fiber-optic tubing on the dental unit.

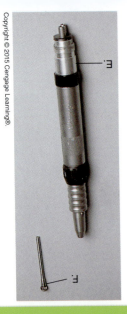

E.

F.

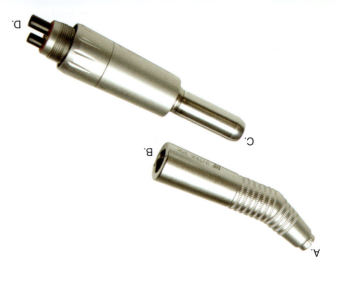

D.

C.

B.

A.

Low-Speed Handpiece

Use

The low-speed handpiece is used in both the dental treatment room and the laboratory. At the dental unit, the low speed is used to polish teeth and restorations, remove soft carious material, and define cavity margins and walls. In the laboratory, the low-speed handpiece is used to trim, smooth, and polish removable dental appliances, such as dentures and partials.

Parts

A. Working end of the low-speed handpiece attachment
B. Connecting end to low-speed motor
C. Low-speed motor that attaches to the connecting end of attachments
D. Low-speed motor that attaches to dental unit and compressed air and water
E. Low-speed handpiece with nose cone
F. Round bur with long shank to be placed in nose cone

Misc.

- Low-speed handpieces operate at or under 30,000 revolutions per minute (rpm).
- The low- or slow-speed handpieces are referred to as the straight handpieces because the shank and head are in a straight line.
- Low-speed handpieces are used with or without attachments. The attachments are either a contra angle or a prophy angle. These attachments are used in the mouth.
- Low-speed handpieces can also be used without attachments. Long-shanked burs are inserted into the working end and used in the dental laboratory.
- Low-speed handpieces and attachments can operate in forward or reverse rotations.
- Low-speed handpieces are to be cleaned or sterilized per the manufacturer's directions.

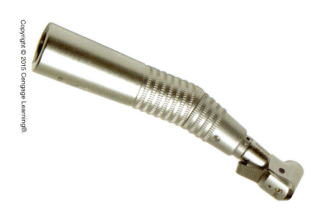

Low-Speed Handpiece with Contra-Angle Attachment

Use	• To hold burs, discs, stones, rubber cups, and brushes for intraoral and extraoral procedures
	• To remove soft decay
	• To polish amalgams
	• To make or finish composite restorations
	• To adjust crowns and bridges
	• To adjust partials and dentures
	• To adjust temporary restorations
Parts	Contra-angle latch attachment on a low-speed handpiece
Misc.	• Uses latch type burs, discs, stones, rubber cups, and brushes

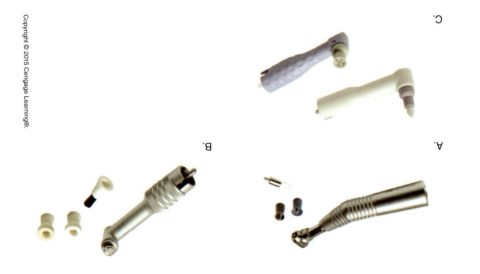

Low-Speed Handpiece with Prophy-Angle Attachment

A.

B.

C.

Use

Parts

- To polish the teeth with rubber cups or brushes

A. Screw-type prophy-angle attachment with screw-type cup and brush
B. Snap-on type prophy-angle attachment with snap-on-type cup and brush
C. Disposable prophy angles with a cup and a brush

Misc.

- Some low-speed handpieces are designed to be lightweight to reduce hand and finger fatigue.
- There are also disposable prophy angles with cups and brushes to attach to low-speed handpieces.

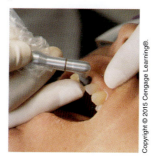

Copyright © 2015 Cengage Learning®.

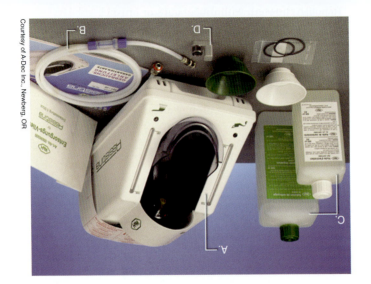

Courtesy of A-Dec Inc., Newberg, OR

Equipment to Clean and Lubricate the Handpieces

Use	To clean and lubricate both high- and low-speed handpieces

Parts

A. Assistina machine
B. Connecting hoses
C. Solutions
D. High-speed adapter

Misc.

- These units must be connected to compressed air.
- They have attachments so both the high- and low-speed handpieces can be run in the same unit.
- Handpieces must be wiped off after the cycle is complete, and then they are ready to be sterilized.
- Several models are available, including the Assistina and the Quatro by Kavo. The manufacturer's directions should be followed.

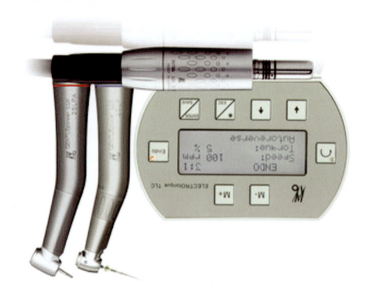

Electric Handpiece

| **Use** | The electric handpiece is used for cavity preparation; endodontic procedures; contouring and trimming provisional crowns and bridges; and adjusting crowns, bridges, and permanent restorations. |

Parts

- Control unit
- Motor and hose
- High-speed attachment with fiber optics
- Low-speed attachment
- Endodontic attachment
- Straight attachment

Misc.

- Electric handpieces are an alternative handpiece to the air-driven handpieces.
- Electric handpieces run from 27,000 to 200,000 rpm.
- Electric handpieces are quiet, vibration free, and efficient.
- Electric handpieces are sterilized.

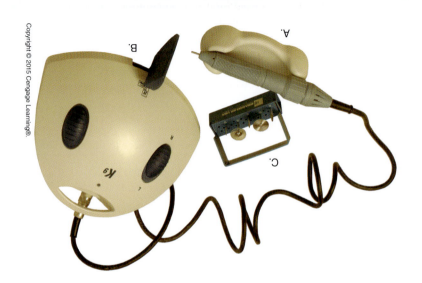

Laboratory Handpiece

Use	• To trim and contour provisional crowns, bridges, and custom trays
	• To adjust and polish partials and dentures
Parts	**A.** Handpiece with holder
	B. Foot control
	C. Selection of burs, stones, and discs
Misc.	• Laboratory handpieces are used for multiple purposes in the dental office.
	• Laboratory handpieces can be used in the reverse or forward direction. The manufacturer's directions should be followed.

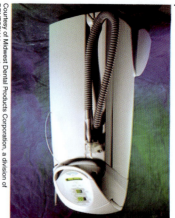

A.

Courtesy of Midwest Dental Products Corporation, a division of DENTSPLY International.

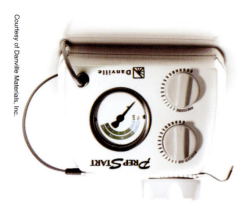

B.

Courtesy of Danville Materials, Inc.

Use	• To clean fissures for sealants
	• To prepare tooth and remove decay in small cavities (example: Class I)
	• To clean restorations
	• To make special repairs in restorations
	• To roughen the inside of restorations before bonding

Use
- To clean fissures for sealants
- To prepare tooth and remove decay in small cavities (example: Class I)
- To clean restorations
- To make special repairs in restorations
- To roughen the inside of restorations before bonding

Parts
- Base unit
- Control panel
- Foot switch
- Air pressure gradient
- Handpiece
- Abrasive flow control
- External suction device

A. Floor model   **B.** Table unit

Misc.
- Each unit requires an air pressure source and abrasive.
- Air abrasion units come in a variety of models, including floor models and countertop units.
- When using air abrasion units, minimal anesthetic is required.
- Abrasive particles are different sizes and made of various materials such as aluminum oxide.
- Abrasive particles must be evacuated when this unit is used, and eye protection must be worn.

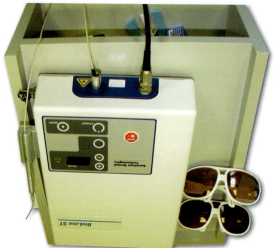

Laser Handpiece

| **Use** | The laser handpiece is used to cut and remove both hard and soft tissue, control bleeding, and biopsy tissue. Dental lasers are also used to cure some dental materials, in cavity preparation and caries removal, in diagnosis transillumination for detection of caries microfractures, in endodontic therapy, in pulpotomy treatment, to whiten teeth, and to treat lesions such as cold sores. |

| **Parts** | Dental laser unit with handpiece attachment and safety glasses |

| **Misc.** | • The dental laser is a medical device that generates a precise beam of concentrated light energy. |
| | • With technology constantly improving, there are many types of dental lasers. |

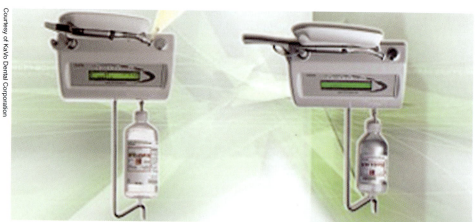

Courtesy of KaVo Dental Corporation

Surgical Unit with Light for Implant Systems

Use	Precise surgical placement of implants, extractions, and oral surgery procedures
Parts	<ul><li>Motor and tubing</li><li>Speed control</li><li>Surgical unit with memory chip</li><li>Irrigation–hygienic unit</li><li>Contra angle with light</li></ul>
Misc.	<ul><li>Sterile water is utilized with the handpiece for cooling.</li><li>Surgical handpieces come with a light.</li><li>Surgical handpieces are electrical and run from a lower speed (used for implants) of 10–50 revolutions per minute (rpms) to a maximum speed of 40,000 rpms.</li><li>Displays actual speed and torque</li></ul>

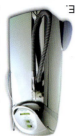

E.

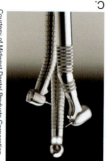

C.

B.

D.

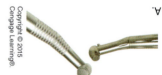

A.

_____ 1. This handpiece is used to rapidly cut tooth structure and finish restorations.

_____ 2. This handpiece is used extraorally to trim and contour provisionals, polish partials and dentures, and to make adjustments to crowns, bridges, and inlays and onlays.

_____ 3. This handpiece has a fiber-optic system that illuminates the area the dentist is working on.

_____ 4. This is a slow-speed handpiece with a contra-angle attachment.

_____ 5. This handpiece requires air and an abrasive to prepare small cavities and clean restorations.

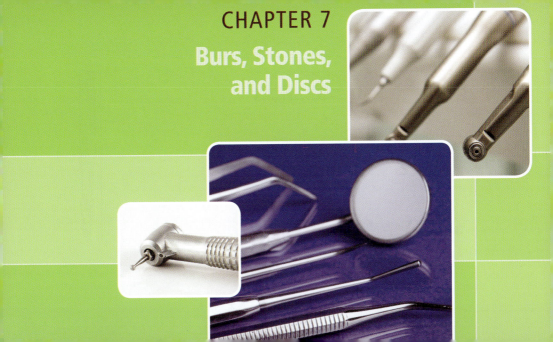

CHAPTER 7

Burs, Stones, and Discs

Burs

Straight shank

Latch-type shank

Friction-grip shank

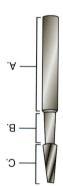

A.

B.

C.

| **Use** | Burs are part of a group of instruments referred to as rotary instruments that cut or polish tooth structure. They are used with high- or low-speed handpieces. Burs are used in numerous laboratory functions. |

Use

Burs are part of a group of instruments referred to as rotary instruments that cut or polish tooth structure. They are used with high- or low-speed handpieces. Burs are used in numerous laboratory functions.

Parts

A. The shank is the part that is inserted into the handpiece.
B. The neck is the tapered connection of the shank to the head.
C. The head is the working end of the bur.

Misc.

- The straight shank, or long shank, functions with the straight, low-speed handpiece.
- The latch-type shank has a notch that fits into the contra-angle/right-angle handpiece and latches securely in place.
- The friction-grip shank functions with the high-speed handpiece.

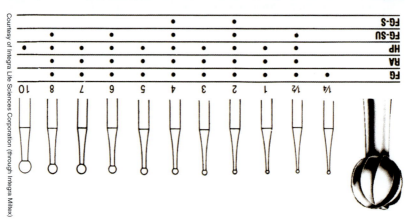

	¼	½	1	2	3	4	5	6	7	8	10	
FG	•	•	•	•	•	•	•	•	•	•	•	
RA		•	•	•	•	•	•	•	•	•	•	
HP		•	•	•	•	•	•	•	•	•	•	•
FG-SU		•	•		•			•		•		
FG-S				•		•						

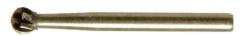

Round Bur

Use	• To open the cavity and remove carious tooth structure
	• To open the tooth for endodontic treatment

Parts	Bladed cutting bur with a shank (friction grip, latch, or straight) and a round cutting head

Misc.	• Available in a range of sizes: 1/4, 1/2, 1, 2, 3, 4, 5, 7, 7, 8, 10
	• The smallest is 1/4, and 10 is the largest.
	• Burs are sterilized and reused until dull and then they are disposed of.

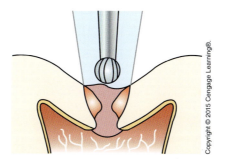

Copyright © 2015 Cengage Learning®.

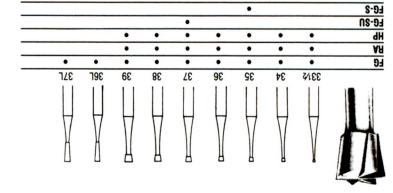

	33½	34	35	36	37	38	39	36L	37L
FG	•	•	•	•	•	•	•	•	•
RA	•	•	•	•	•	•	•		
HP	•	•	•	•	•	•	•		
FG-SU					•				
FG-S				•					

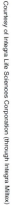

Inverted Cone Bur

| **Use** | • Removes caries |
| | • Makes undercuts in the preparation for retention |

Parts

Bladed cutting bur with a shank (friction grip, latch, or straight) and a short tapered cutting head

Misc.

- Available in a range of sizes: 33 1/2: 34, 35, 37, 37, 38, 39, 37L, 37L
- The smallest is 33 1/2, and 39 is the largest; 37L and 37L have a longer head.
- *L* indicates long head on the bur.
- *S* indicates short head on the bur.
- Burs are sterilized and reused until dull and then they are disposed of.
- Burs are purchased individually in packages or several in one package.

Plain Fissure Straight Bur and Plain Fissure Cross-Cut Bur

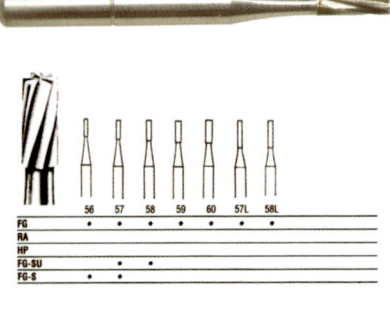

	56	57	58	59	60	57L	58L
FG	•	•	•	•	•	•	•
RA							
HP							
FG-SU		•	•				
FG-S	•	•					

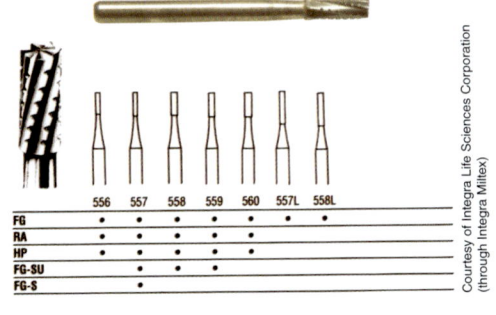

	556	557	558	559	560	557L	558L
FG	•	•	•	•	•	•	•
RA	•	•	•				
HP	•	•	•	•	•		
FG-SU	•	•	•	•			
FG-S		•					

| **Use** | • Forms the cavity walls of the preparation |
| | • Places retention grooves in walls of cavity preparation |

Parts

This is a bladed cutting bur with a shank (friction grip, latch, or straight) and a long straight cutting head. The cross-cut bur has horizontal cuts.

Misc.

- Head has parallel sides (cross-cut with horizontal cutting edges)
- Available in a range of sizes: 57, 57, 58, 59, 70, 57L, 58L (straight) and 557, 557, 558, 559, 557L, 558L (cross-cut)
- *L* indicates long head on the bur.
- *S* indicates short head on the bur.
- Burs are sterilized and reused until dull and then they are disposed of.

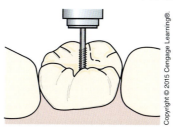

Copyright © 2015 Cengage Learning®.

Tapered Fissure Straight Bur and Tapered Fissure Cross-Cut Bur

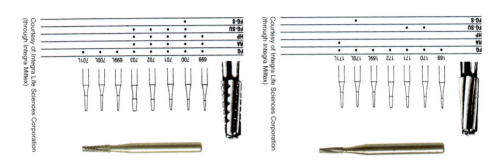

Courtesy of Integra Life Sciences Corporation (through Integra Miltex)

Courtesy of Integra Life Sciences Corporation (through Integra Miltex)

Use

- Forms divergent walls (angles) of the cavity preparation
- Places retention grooves in the walls of the cavity preparation

Parts

This is a bladed cutting bur with a shank (friction grip, latch, or straight) and a long tapered cutting head.

Misc.

- Available in a range of sizes: 179, 170, 171, 172, 179L, 170L, 171L (straight) and 799, 700, 701, 702, 703, 799L, 700L, 701L (cross-cut)
- *L* indicates long head on the bur.
- *S* indicates short head on the bur.
- Burs are sterilized and reused until dull and then they are disposed of
- The head of the cross-cut bur is tapered and has horizontal cutting edges.

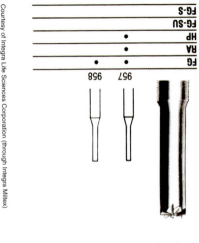

	FG	RA	HP	FG-SU	FG-S
957	•	•	•		
958	•		•		

End-Cutting Bur

Use

Forms the shoulder for crown preparations

Parts

A cutting bur with a shank (friction grip, latch, or straight); only bladed on the end of a cylinder head

Misc.

- Range of sizes: 957, 958
- Burs are sterilized until dull and then they are disposed of.

							FG-S
							FG-SU
		•					HP
		•					RA
		•					FG

14

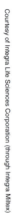

Wheel

Use	Forms retention in preparations, often used in Class V preparations
Parts	A bladed cutting bur with a shank (friction grip, latch, or straight) and wheel-shaped short head
Misc.	<ul><li>The head has cutting edges on the top and the sides.</li><li>Size: 14</li><li>Burs are sterilized until dull and then they are disposed of.</li></ul>

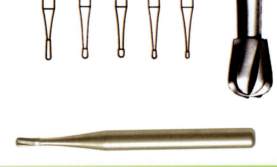

	FG	RA	HP	FG-SU	FG-S
329	•				
330	•				•
331	•				
332	•				
331L	•				

Courtesy of Integra Life Sciences Corporation (through Integra Miltex)

Pear Bur

Use	• Opens and extends the cavity preparation
	• Removes dental decay

Parts   This is a bladed cutting bur with a shank (friction grip, latch, or straight) and a pear-shaped head.

Misc.
- The head of the bur is shaped like a pear, with the largest part away from the neck of the bur.
- The bur has cutting edges on all sides of the head.
- Common range of sizes: 329, 330, 331, 332, 331L
- *L* indicates long head on the bur.
- *S* indicates short head on the bur.
- Burs are sterilized and reused until dull and then they are disposed of.

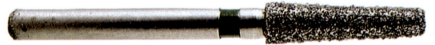

Courtesy of Midwest Dental Products Corporation, a division of DENTSPLY International.

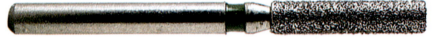

Courtesy of Midwest Dental Products Corporation, a division of DENTSPLY International.

Diamond Bur Flat-End Taper and Flat-End Cylinder

<table>
<tr><td>

Use

</td><td>

- Rapid reduction of tooth for crown preparation when a square shoulder is needed (taper) or when parallel wall and flat preparation floor is needed (cylinder)
- Rapid reduction of tooth for crown preparation

</td></tr>
<tr><td>

Parts

</td><td>

The head of the diamond bur is embedded with diamond particles through an electroplating or a bonding process.

</td></tr>
<tr><td>

Misc.

</td><td>

- Variety of shapes, sizes, and grits
- Superfine is used to finish restorations.
- Grit is designated by the color band on the shank of the diamond bur or by the letter after the name of the diamond bur.
- Burs are sterilized and reused until dull and then they are disposed of.

</td></tr>
</table>

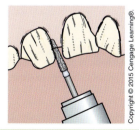

Copyright © 2015 Cengage Learning®.

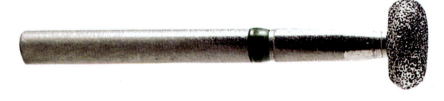

Diamond Bur Flame and Diamond Bur Wheel

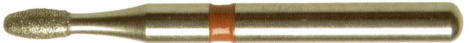

Use
- Rapid reduction of tooth for crown preparation when a beveled subgingival margin is needed (flame)
- Rapid reduction of the incisal edge during crown preparation (wheel)
- Rapid reduction of the lingual aspect of the anterior teeth during crown preparation (wheel)

Parts
The head of the diamond bur is embedded with diamond particles through an electroplating or bonding process.

Misc.
- Variety of shapes, sizes, and grits
- The flame shape can be short, as shown, or long and tapered.
- Superfine is used to finish restorations.
- The wheel is sometimes called a donut shape.
- Burs are sterilized and reused until dull and then they are disposed of.

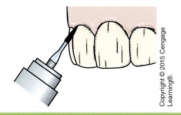

Copyright © 2015 Cengage Learning®.

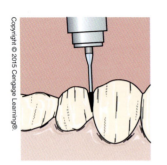

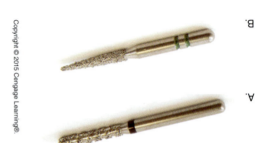

B.

A.

Diamond Turbo or Speed Cut and Diamond Composite Finishing Bur

Use	• Rapid cutting and gross reduction of the tooth structure
	• Used to finish composite restorations
	• Used to finish glass ionomer and porcelain restorations
Parts	• Cross-cuts or spiral cuts on head of diamond bur; head is embedded with diamond particles through an electroplating or bonding process.
	A. Spiral shape
	B. Dual-cross
Misc.	• Variety of shapes with cross-cuts or spiral cuts in the diamond head
	• Diamonds are designed with diamond-free cooling zones that absorb normal heat production.
	• Burs are sterilized and reused until dull and then they are disposed of.
	• Available from ultra-fine to extra-coarse grits
	• Superfine is used to finish restorations.
	• Available in long and short shanks

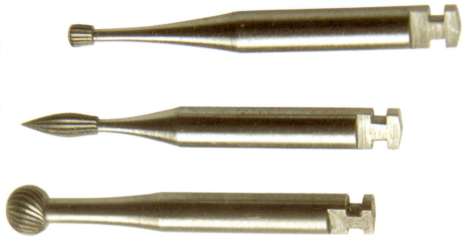

Finishing Bur

Use	• To smooth, trim, and finish metal restorations
	• To smooth, trim, and finish natural-tooth-colored material restorations
Parts	Up to 30 or more blades for ultra-fine finishing
Misc.	• Variety of shapes and sizes
	• Identified by the manufacturer's number
	• Available in latch (as shown) and friction grip
	• Burs are sterilized until dull and then they are disposed of.

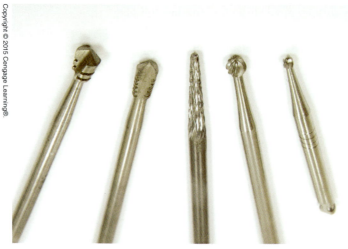

Surgical Bur

Use	Used in low-speed handpiece to reduce and contour the alveolar bone and tooth structure
Parts	<ul><li>Extra-long shanked bur in many shapes to allow for access</li><li>The head is designed to cut tooth or bone structure.</li></ul>
Misc.	<ul><li>Heads come in various sizes and shapes.</li><li>Long shanks</li><li>Burs are sterilized until dull and then they are disposed of.</li></ul>

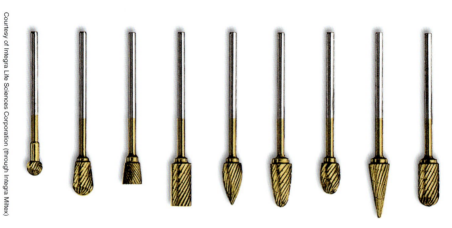

Laboratory Burs

Laboratory burs are sometimes referred to as vulcanite burs.

Use
- To make adjustments on acrylic materials, such as partials, dentures, and custom trays
- Used on plaster, stone, and metal materials

Parts
- Long shanks insert into straight low-speed handpieces.
- Large working ends

Misc.
- Variety of sizes and shapes
- Available in titanium-nitrate-coated carbide
- Titanium-nitrate-coated burs are faster, cooler, and longer lasting

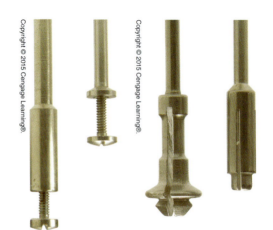

Mandrel Snap-On and Mandrel Screw-On

| Use | • Used with different abrasives that are mounted to the rods |
| | • Used to hold the discs that finish and polish |

Use
- Used with different abrasives that are mounted to the rods
- Used to hold the discs that finish and polish

Parts

Rods of various lengths that are used in low-speed handpieces with snap-on or screw-on attachments

Misc.
- Short-shank snap-on or screw-on mandrel used with contra-angle slow-speed handpiece
- Long shank used with straight slow-speed handpiece
- Available in friction grip
- Can be sterilized or available in disposable types

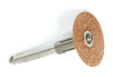

A.

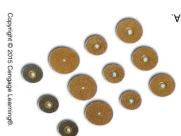

Sandpaper Discs

| **Use** | • To polish, smooth, and adjust restorative materials |
| | • To polish, smooth, and adjust dental appliances |

Parts	• Circular discs
	• Abrasive texture on one or both sides
	• Mounted to mandrel for use

A. Sandpaper discs
B. Soft sandpaper discs in various sizes and grits
C. Snap on garnet disc attached to mandrel

Misc.	• Can be rigid or flexible
	• Available in a variety of sizes and grits
	• When ordering, the size, grit, abrasiveness, and type of mandrel must be specified.

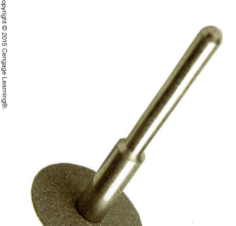
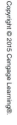
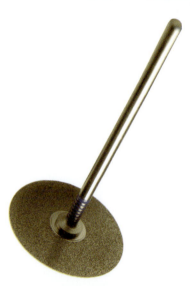

Diamond Disc

Use	• Rapid cutting
	• Polishing composite restorations
	• Interproximal reduction
Parts	Circular steel discs
Misc.	• Available in solid discs or patterned discs
	• Discs have diamond particles or chips bonded to both sides of steel discs.
	• Discs are sterilized and reused until dull and then they are disposed of.

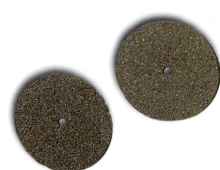

Carborundum Discs

Use	• Used primarily in the dental laboratory to cut and finish gold restorations
	• Can be used intra-orally
	• Used for trimming acrylic provisional restorations
Parts	• Circular, thin, brittle discs that break easily
	• Carborundum on both sides
	• Mounted to a mandrel
Misc.	• Called separating discs
	• Discs are disposed of.
	• Carborundum discs are also known as Jo-dandy discs.

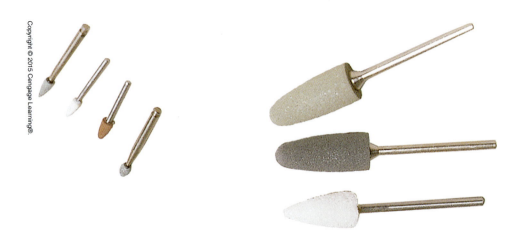

Rubber Points

Use	To polish restorations
Parts	• Rubber-tip head that is impregnated with abrasive material
	• Latch-type or friction-grip shanks
Misc.	• White points are for polishing.
	• Green points (greenies) are not as abrasive as brown points.
	• Brown points (brownies) are more abrasive than green points.

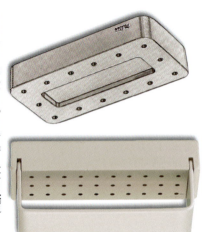

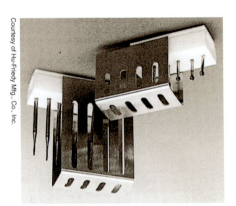

Bur Blocks

On dental tray setups

Holding device for burs

- Variety of shapes, sizes, and manufacturers
- Most can be sterilized.
- Holds both friction-grip and latch-type burs
- Some are magnetic to hold burs in place.

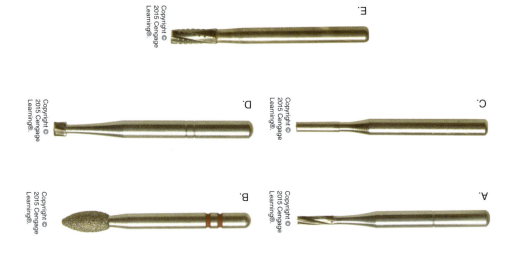

E.

D.

C.

B.

A.

Test Your Knowledge

_____ 1. Identify the plain fissure straight bur.
_____ 2. Identify the inverted cone bur.
_____ 3. Identify the plain fissure cross-cut bur.
_____ 4. Identify the diamond bur.
_____ 5. Identify the end-cutting bur.

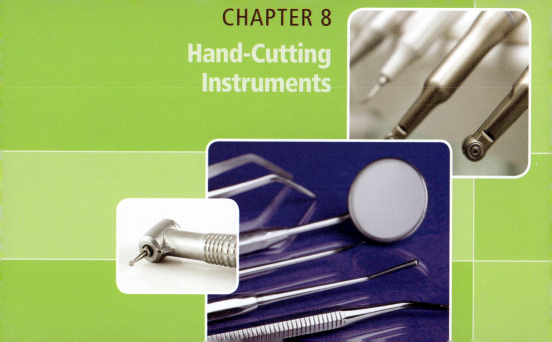

CHAPTER 8

Hand-Cutting Instruments

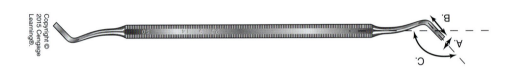

A.

B.

C.

Black's formula was developed by G. V. Black to standardize the exact size and angulation of an instrument. Black's formula for three-number hand-cutting instruments includes the length and width of the blade and the angle at which the blade is positioned to the handle. These numbers are found on the handle of chisels, hatchets, and hoes.

Three-Number Formula

A. The width of the blade in tenths of a millimeter. In the formula 20-9-14, the 20 indicates the blade is 2.0 mm wide.
B. The length of the blade in millimeters. The 9 indicates that the blade is 9 mm long.
C. The angle of the blade to the long axis of the handle in degrees centigrade. The 14 indicates that the instrument has a blade at an angle of 14/100 of a circle.

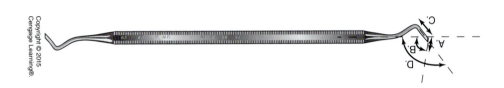

Black's formula for four-number hand-cutting instruments includes the length and width of the blade, the angle at which the blade is positioned to the handle, and the angle of the cutting edge of the blade to the handle. These numbers are found on the handle of angle formers and gingival margin trimmers.

Four-Number Formula

A. The width of the blade in tenths of a millimeter. In the formula 15-85-8-12, the 15 indicates the blade is 1.5 mm long.

B. This number is added to make the four-number formula. It is the degree of the angle of the cutting edge of the blade to the handle of the instrument. The 85 indicates that the cutting edge forms an 85-degree C angle with the handle.

C. The length of the blade in millimeters. The 8 indicates that the blade is 8 mm long.

D. The angle of the blade to the long axis of the handle. The 12 indicates the blade forms a 12-degree C angle with the handle of the instrument.

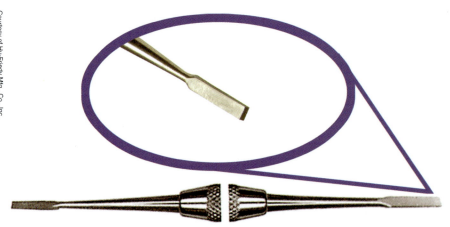

Straight Chisel

Use	• To shape and plane enamel and dentin walls of the cavity preparation
	• Used in a pushing action
	• Used in Class II or IV cavity preparations
	• Used with a mallet to remove crowns
Parts	• Straight-shanked instrument with bevel on one side of the cutting edge
	• Single or double ended
Misc.	• Single or double ended
	• Needs to be sharpened
	• This is a three-number instrument.

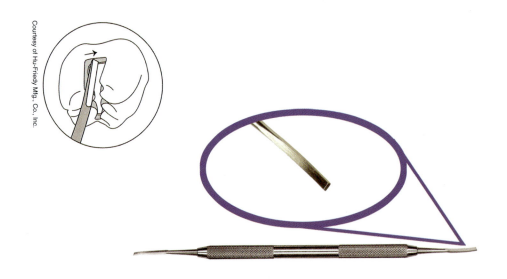

Courtesy of Hu-Friedy Mfg., Co., Inc.

Wedelstaedt Chisel

Use	
	• To shape and plane enamel and dentin walls of the cavity preparation
	• Used in a pushing action
	• Used for Class III and IV cavity preparations
Parts	• Slightly curved blade on a shanked instrument with bevel on one side of the cutting edge
	• Single or double ended
Misc.	• Single or double ended
	• This is a three-number instrument.

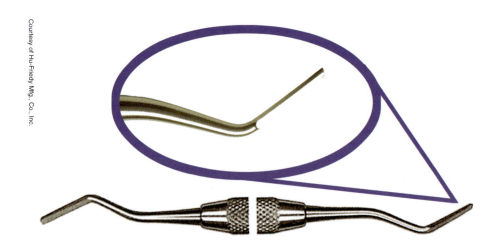

Binangle Chisel

Use
- To shape and plane enamel and dentin walls of the cavity preparation
- Used in a pushing action
- Used in a Class II cavity preparation

Parts

Has two angles in the shank of the instrument

Misc.
- Usually a double-ended instrument
- This is a three-number instrument.

Hatchets

Use	• To refine the cavity walls and to obtain retention in the cavity preparation
	• Used in a downward motion
Parts	• Paired left and right with the bevel on one side of the blade on one end of the instrument and on the reverse side of the blade on the other end
Misc.	• Usually a double-ended instrument
	• Sometimes referred to as an enamel hatchet
	• This is a three-number instrument.

Hoes

Use
- To smooth and shape the floor of the cavity preparation
- Used in a pulling motion

Parts
- A shank and head shaped similar to a garden hoe with straight and angled shanks

Misc.
- The cutting edge of the blade is nearly perpendicular to the shank/handle.
- Is a three-number instrument
- Is normally single ended

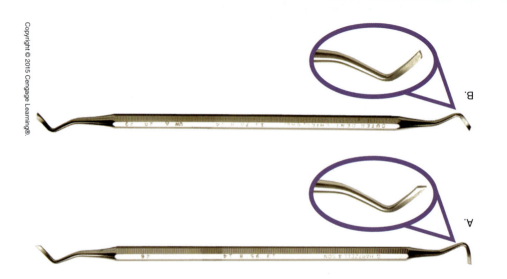

B.

A.

Gingival Margin Trimmers

Use

To bevel the gingival margin wall of the cavity preparation

Parts

- A pair of instruments with binangled shanks used to smooth the mesial and distal cervical margins of the cavity preparation
- The blade is curved instead of being straight. One end curves to the right; the other curves to the left.
- The cutting edge is slanted.

A. Distal gingival margin trimmer (GMT)

- Close-up of the working end of the distal GMT

B. Mesial gingival margin trimmer

- Close-up of the working end of the mesial GMT

Misc.

- A pair of (GMTs) is used during the cavity preparation because one instrument is used for the distal surfaces (A) and another is for the mesial surface (B).
- This is a four-numbered instrument. If the second number of the four-number formula is 90 or above, it is used on the distal surface of the cavity preparation. If it is 85 or below, it is used on the mesial surface.

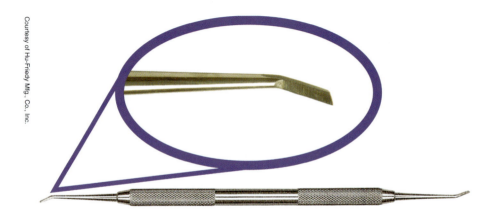

Angle Formers

Use
To form and define point angles and to sharpen line angles in a cavity preparation

Parts
This is a double-ended instrument where the cutting edge is slanted and ends in a point. The slanted cutting edge is beveled differently on each end of the instrument to allow access to the mesial and distal surfaces of the cavity preparation.

Misc.
- Four-number instrument
- Usually a double-ended instrument

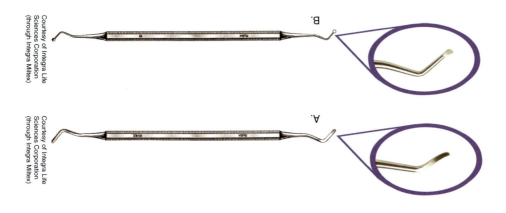

A.

Courtesy of Integra Life
Sciences Corporation
(through Integra Miltex)

B.

Courtesy of Integra Life
Sciences Corporation
(through Integra Miltex)

Excavators—Spoon and Blade Excavators

Use	• To remove carious materials and debris from the teeth
	• To assist in the tucking/inverting of the dental dam around the teeth
	• To remove temporary crowns and bridges during fabrication
	• To remove excess temporary cement from around the temporary restorations
Parts	• A bladed instrument with a binangled shank that is rounded at the working end of the blade
	A. Blade excavator
	B. Spoon excavator
Misc.	• Ends are spoon shaped with cutting edges.
	• Single and double ended
	• Ends vary in size.

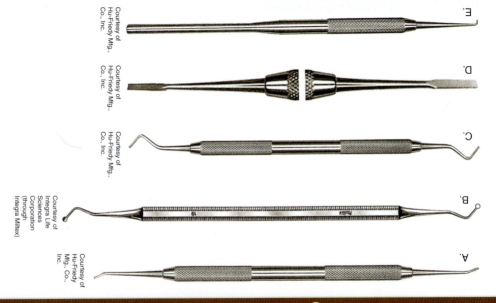

E.

Courtesy of
Hu-Friedy Mfg.,
Co., Inc.

D.

Courtesy of
Hu-Friedy Mfg.,
Co., Inc.

C.

Courtesy of
Hu-Friedy Mfg.,
Co., Inc.

B.

Courtesy of
Integra Life
Sciences
Corporation
(through
Integra Miltex)

A.

Courtesy of
Hu-Friedy
Mfg., Co.,
Inc.

_____ 1. This hand-cutting instrument is used in a downward motion to refine the walls of the cavity preparation.

_____ 2. This hand-cutting instrument is used in a pushing action to shape and plane the walls of the cavity preparation and has a straight shank.

_____ 3. This hand-cutting instrument is used to remove carious material and debris from the tooth.

_____ 4. This hand-cutting instrument is used in a pulling motion to smooth and shape the floor of the cavity preparation.

_____ 5. This instrument is an "angle former."

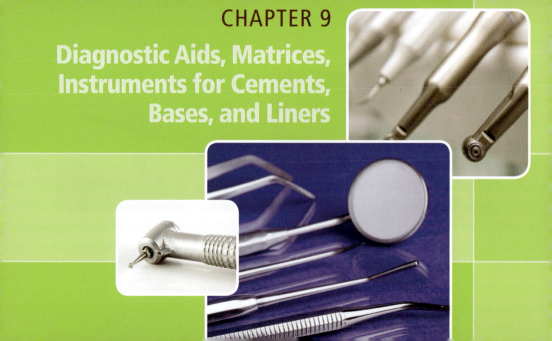

CHAPTER 9

Diagnostic Aids, Matrices, Instruments for Cements, Bases, and Liners

Intraoral Camera

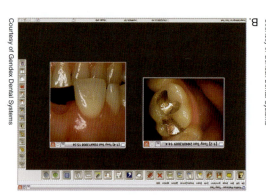

A.

Courtesy of Gendex Dental Systems

B.

Courtesy of Gendex Dental Systems

Use	• Allows patients to see areas and conditions inside their mouths while the dentist is discussing them
	• To take photos that can be saved in patients' electronic records or printed for their paper records
	• Used for marketing, patient presentation, and helping the patient understand needed treatment
Parts	Handheld wand with camera that takes intraoral pictures and is attached to the unit and computer terminal
Misc.	• Allows the office to be paperless
	• May be attached to the unit or a mobile unit
	• Can be used by the dentist or auxiliary
	• Barriers are used on the wand
	• The systems are designed to obtain different views of the tooth/teeth for better diagnosis.

A.

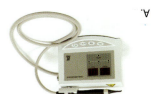

B.

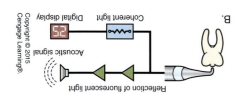

Digital display

Coherent light

Acoustic signal

Reflection of fluorescent light

C.

Courtesy of KaVo Dental Corporation

Use	• To detect carious material in the tooth
	• To ensure that the tooth is free of caries prior to sealant placement
	• To quantify caries progression

Use
- To detect carious material in the tooth
- To ensure that the tooth is free of caries prior to sealant placement
- To quantify caries progression

Parts
- Available as a battery-operated microprocessor-controlled display unit with handpiece and tips or a handheld pen unit with tips for easier handling and greater mobility

A. Kavo DIAGNOdent unit
B. How caries detection works
C. Close-up of the handheld pen unit

Misc.
- Tips are to be sterilized.
- Lasers may also emit audio signals.
- A decayed tooth structure and bacteria fluoresce (give off light) when exposed to specific wavelengths of light. Thus a healthy tooth exhibits little or no fluorescence, whereas a tooth with decay fluoresces according to the extent of decay.

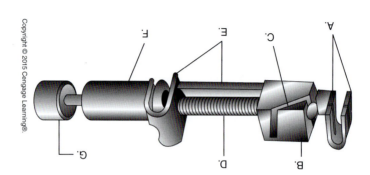

A.

B.

C.

D.

E.

F.

G.

Copyright © 2015 Cengage Learning®.

| **Use** | To hold the matrix band that establishes the normal contour of the prepared tooth while the tooth is being filled with the restorative material |

| **Parts** | **A.** Guide channels: The slots in the end of the retainer that hold the matrix band. The slots direct the band to the right or left of the retainer. |

B. Vise (locking): Holds the ends of the matrix band in place in the diagonal slots.

C. Diagonal slot: Where the matrix band is placed. This part slides up and down on the spindle.

D. Spindle: A screw-like rod used to secure the band in the vise.

E. Frame: The main body of the retainer.

F. Inner knob (adjusting knob): Used to adjust the size of the matrix band loop by moving the vise along the frame of the retainer.

G. Outer knob (locking knob): Used to tighten and loosen the spindle against the band in the vise.

Matrix Bands

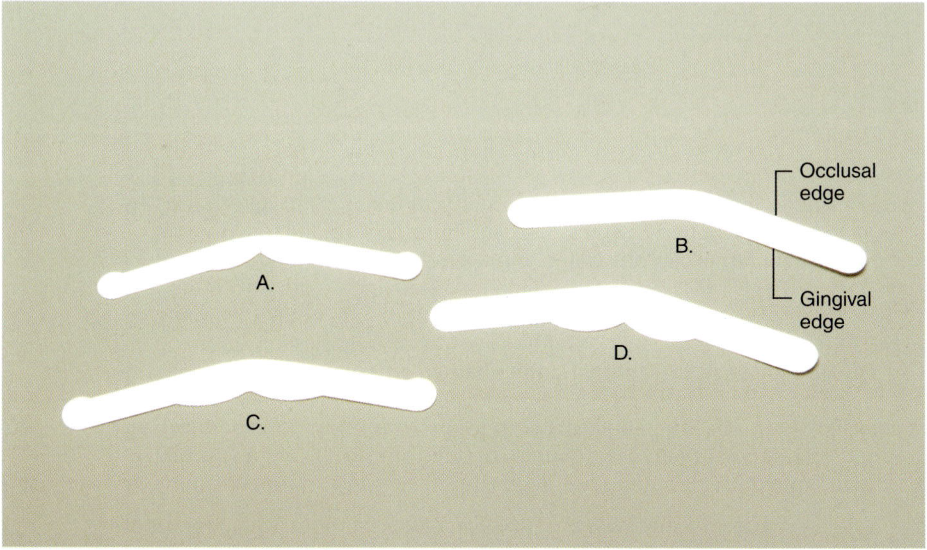

C.

D.

Gingival edge

B.

Occlusal edge

A.

Use   Forms the missing surface or wall and reestablishes the normal contour of the prepared tooth while the tooth is being filled with the restorative material

Parts
A. Pediatric band used for primary teeth
B. Universal band
   • Occlusal edge
   • Gingival edge
C. Premolar band
D. Molar band

Misc.
• Matrix bands are made of stainless steel.
• Matrix bands are normally the same length.
• Matrix bands differ in the shape of one edge and in their widths.
• The size of the cavity prep indicates which band is used.

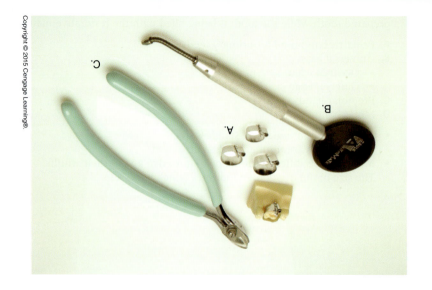

A.

B.

C.

Auto-Matrix Kit

Use	Forms the missing surface or wall and reestablishes the normal contour of the prepared tooth while the tooth is being filled with the restorative material
Parts	**A.** Matrix and coil: Used to loop the tooth and replace the missing surface or tooth wall
	B. Tightening device and rotation handle: Used to tighten the matrix around the tooth; it fits into the coil and tightens as the handle is rotated.
	C. Removal pliers: Used to clip the end of the auto-lock loop
Misc.	• The stainless steel bands are conical shaped and come in four sizes.
	• The matrix and coil (bands) are circles with auto-lock loops that lock the matrices on the teeth.
	• There is no retainer to obstruct the operator's access or vision.

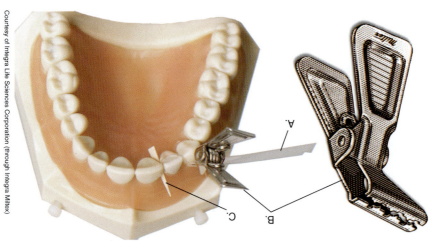

Courtesy of Integra Life Sciences Corporation (through Integra Miltex)

A.

B.

C.

Plastic Strip Matrix

Use
- Provide anatomical contour and proximal contact relation to the tooth
- Prevent excess material at the gingival margin
- Confine the restorative material under pressure while the material is being cured
- Protect the restorative material from losing or gaining moisture during the setting time
- Allow the polymerizing light to reach the composite restorative material

Parts
A. Strip matrix
B. Clip retainer
C. Wedge

Misc.
- Used with composite, glass ionomer, or compomer restorative materials on anterior teeth
- Made of nylon, acetate, celluloid, or resin
- Approximately 3 inches long and 3/8 inch wide

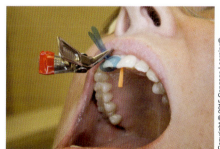

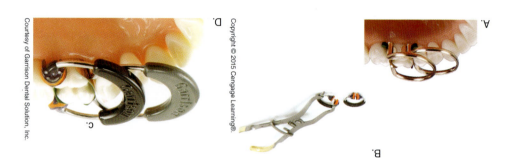

A.

B.

C.

D.

Sectional Matrix System

Use	Sectional matrix rings that confine the restorative material under pressure while the material is being cured
Parts	**A.** G-rings (to hold the matrix tightly in place) **B.** Ring placement forceps (hinged forceps that are designed to fit the g-rings and securely grasp the rings) **C.** Oval matrix bands **D.** Sectional matrix system in place for mesio-occluso-distal (MOD) restoration
Misc.	• Bands are available in different sizes and shapes to accommodate restorations, including adult and pediatric bands and extended bands for deep cervical restorations.

Wedges and Wedge Wands

A.

B.

C.

Wedge Wands

Use	• To tightly hold matrix band in place along the gingival margins of Class II, III, and IV preparations
	• To prevent excess filling material from escaping between the tooth and the matrix band
	• To ensure good contact with the adjacent tooth after the band has been removed

Parts
- Small, triangular piece of wood or plastic
- **A.** Sample of wooden wedges
- **B.** Sample of light cure-through wedges
- **C.** Wedge wands: the wand is one-piece flexible plastic wedge that separates after application.

Misc.
- Variety of shapes and sizes available
- Either natural, clear, or colored
- Usually come in an assortment kit with various sizes
- Colors mark the different sizes within the kit.
- Can come in flexible, curved, or with attached sectional matrix
- The difference between the wedges and the wedge wands is the detachable handle. Removal of the wedge from the wand is done by applying gentle force on the waffle-like neck of the wand.
- Available in cure-through

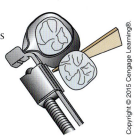

| Use | • To place and condense pliable restorative materials |
| | • To place cement bases in the cavity preparation |

Parts	• Usually double ended
	• Paddle end to place materials
	• Small condenser end or different-shaped paddle end

| Misc. | • Available in various sizes, angles, and shapes |
| | • Used for placement of intermediate and temporary materials |

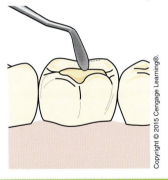

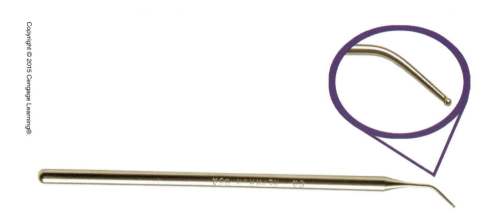

Small-Balled Instrument (Dycal Instrument)

Use	Mix and place two-paste calcium hydroxide material or glass ionomer liner into the cavity preparation
Parts	• Small-balled tip • Straight handle
Misc.	• Also called a liner applicator or dycal instrument • Available in short or long handle

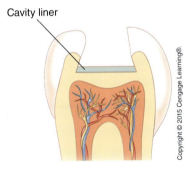

Cavity liner

Copyright © 2015 Cengage Learning®.

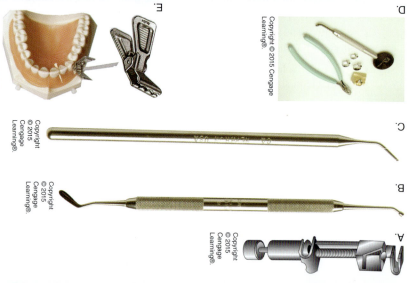

A.
Copyright © 2015 Cengage Learning®.

B.
Copyright © 2015 Cengage Learning®.

C.
Copyright © 2015 Cengage Learning®.

D.
Copyright © 2015 Cengage Learning®.

E.
Courtesy of Integra Life Sciences Corporation (through Integra Miltex)

_____ 1. Identify the Tofflemire matrix.
_____ 2. Identify the sectional matrix system.
_____ 3. Identify the strip matrix.
_____ 4. Identify the plastic filling instrument.
_____ 5. Identify the instrument used to mix and place liners.

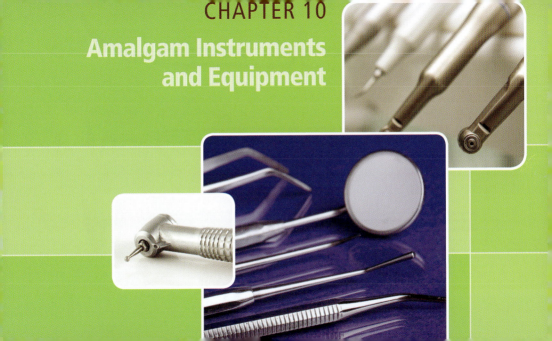

CHAPTER 10

Amalgam Instruments and Equipment

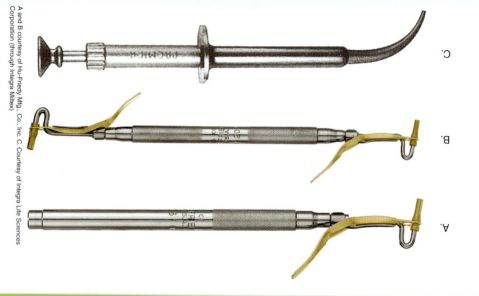

Amalgam Carriers

A.

B.

C.

Use	To carry and dispense amalgam into the cavity preparation; the back-action condenser
Parts	• An instrument with a hollow tube on one end that amalgam is placed into and then dispensed into the cavity prep with a spring action

A. May be single ended
B. May be double ended
C. An amalgam gun is a single-ended carrier made of high-grade plastic or metal.

Misc.	• Double-ended carriers have a small and large end.
	• Most carriers are made of stainless steel; some have Teflon or coated barrels to prevent clogging.

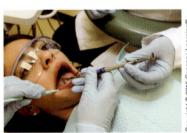

Copyright © 2015 Cengage Learning®.

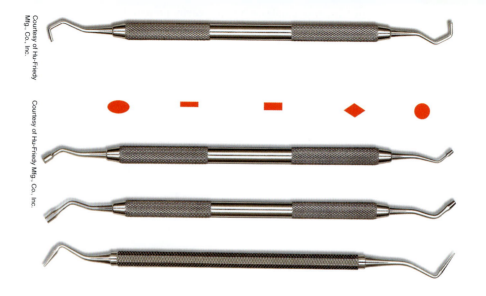

Amalgam Condensers and Back-Action Condensers

Use	To pack and condense amalgam into the cavity preparation; back-action gets in difficult-to-reach areas
Parts	• An instrument that has an end similar to a hammer that packs the amalgam into the preparation • Single or double ended
Misc.	• Condensers are diverse in design to be functional in the locations and designs of cavity preparations. • Working ends may be plain (smooth) or serrated. • Sometimes called "pluggers" • Double-ended condensers have one small end and one large end. • Variety of shapes of the working ends: round, diamond, rectangular, and ovoid condenser (shown in red) • The shank has three angles. • Double and single ended

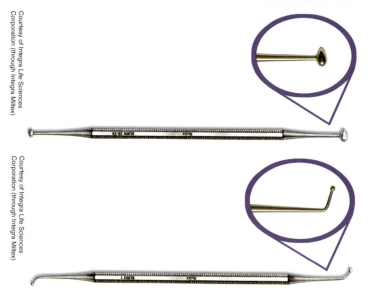

Ball Burnisher and Football Burnisher

| **Use** | • To smooth rough margins of restoration |
| | • To shape metal matrix bands |

Parts

An instrument that has a rounded ball tip or a football-shaped tip used to smooth materials that are in the preparation

Misc.

• Double or single ended
• On the double-ended ball or football burnisher, the ends may be different sizes.

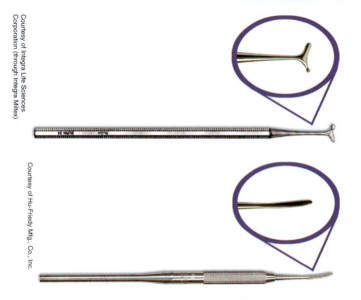

Beavertail Burnisher and T-Ball Burnisher

Courtesy of Integra Life Sciences
Corporation (through Integra Miltex)

Courtesy of Hu-Friedy Mfg., Co., Inc.

Use	• To smooth rough margins of amalgam restorations
	• To shape metal matrix bands
	• The beavertail is used to tuck or invert the dental dam material around the teeth.
	• The T-ball is used to slightly separate the teeth when contacts are very tight.
Parts	• An instrument that has a flat beavertail-shaped tip used to smooth materials that are in the preparation
	• An instrument that has a T-shaped end with a ball on one extension and a blade on the other used to smooth materials that are in the preparation
Misc.	• Double or single ended
	• The T-ball burnisher comes in different sizes and is single ended.

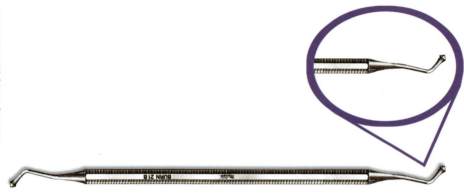

Courtesy of Integra Life Sciences Corporation
(through Integra Miltex)

Acorn Burnisher

Use	• To smooth amalgam after placement
	• To begin carving of amalgam restoration by placing the initial grooves
Parts	An instrument that has an acorn-shaped end used to smooth materials that are in the preparation
Misc.	• Single or double ended
	• On double-ended acorn ball burnishers, the ends may be different sizes.
	• Can be used for composites as well

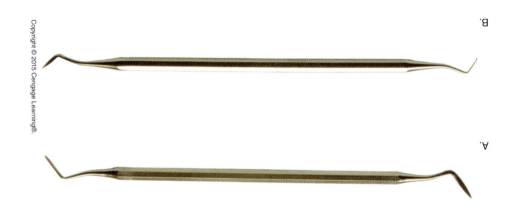

B.

A.

Hollenback Carver and Half-Hollenback Carver

| **Use** | • To remove excess restorative material
• To carve occlusal anatomy
• To carve interproximal anatomy |

| **Parts** | **A.** Hollenback carver
B. Half-Hollenback carver (same shape blades as the Hollenback carver, just smaller in size) |

| **Misc.** | • Double ended: working ends positioned at different angles
• Available in different sizes |

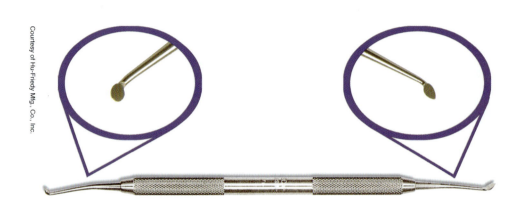

Cleoid-Discoid Carver

Use	• To remove excess restorative material
	• To carve and shape the occlusal anatomy
Parts	• Double-ended instrument with two different ends
	• Cleoid end: looks like a claw or a spade and is pointed
	• Discoid end: round end; looks like a disc
Misc.	• Places the pits, fissures, and the anatomy in the restoration
	• If the bite is high, it is used to reduce the restoration material.

T-3 Carver

Use	• To remove excess restorative material
	• To carve and shape the occlusal anatomy
Parts	Double ended: One end is shaped like a disc and the other end is a blade.
Misc.	• Places the pits, fissures, and the anatomy in the restoration
	• If the bite is high, it is used to reduce the restoration material.
	• Has the function of two different instruments in one

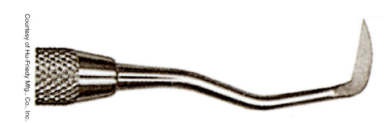

Gold Carving Knife

Use	• To trim excess filling material in the interproximal surfaces
	• To shape the contour of the tooth interproximal
Parts	An instrument that has two or three angles in the shank that ends in a sharp knife blade; the ends appear at different angles.
Misc.	• Single and double ended
	• Variety of shapes and designs
	• Sometimes referred to as a gold finishing knife
	• Also used with composite restorative material

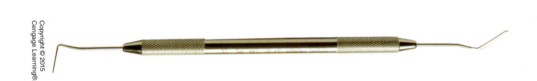

Interproximal Carver (IPC) Instrument

- To trim excess filling material in the interproximal surfaces
- To carve and smooth interproximal surfaces

An instrument with long thin blades on each end placed at different angles

- Variety of shapes and designs
- Single or double ended
- Thin blade aids in getting into the interproximal area to carve
- Also used with composite restorative material

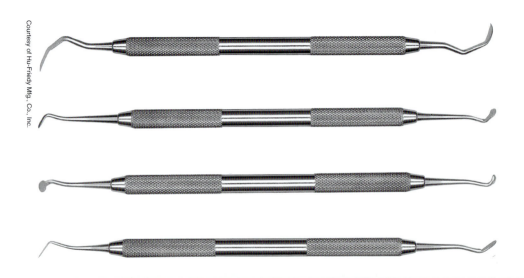

Tanner Carver

Use	To carve and shape the occlusal anatomy of an amalgam restoration
Parts	An instrument with many different types of shapes on the working ends used to carve the occlusal anatomy
Misc.	• Doubled-ended instrument
	• The two ends are different shapes, such as a spade on one end and a disc on the other.
	• The ends may also be configured as a blade with each end at a different angle.

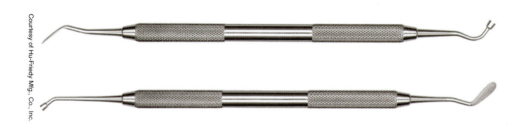

Woodson Plastic Filling Instrument

Use	• To pass and place (condense) various dental materials during cavity preparation
	• To place temporary restorative materials into cavity preparation
Parts	A double-ended instrument that has a condenser on one end and a blade on the other
Misc.	• Comes in a variety of sizes and some variation of shapes
	• The angle of the blade may be rotated.

A.

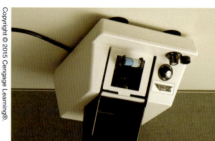

B.

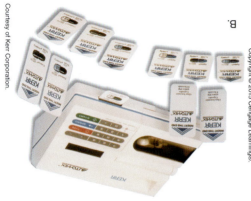

Use	• Mechanical means to combine dental alloy and mercury into dental amalgam: restorative material
	• To mix various pre-capsulated dental cements, both permanent and temporary
Parts	• Equipment that comes with cradles to hold amalgam capsules, cradle cover, a timer, and speed control
	A. Dental amalgamator with manual controls
	B. Dental amalgamator with programmable computerized mixing system
Misc.	• Amalgam capsules contain dental alloy, mercury, a membrane separating the two components, and a pestle to mix the amalgam.
	• Capsules are placed in a cradle (some have to be twisted or pushed to activate), and the cover is closed before beginning.
	• The process of mixing is also called trituration or amalgamation.
	• Follow the manufacturer's directions for time and speed settings.

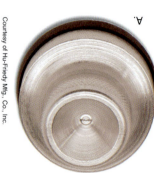

A.

B.

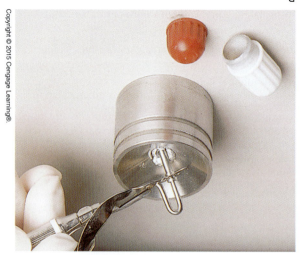

| **Use** | • To hold the pliable amalgam just after trituration |
| | • To load the amalgam into the carrier |

Parts Metal or glass dished-out containers designed for easy use with the amalgam carrier

A. Metal Amalgam well
B. Placing the Amalgam into the carrier from the amalgam well

Misc.
- Different shapes and designs
- Can be sterilized if there is not a foam pad on the bottom

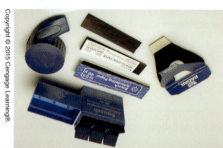

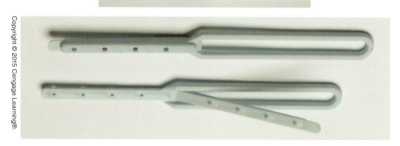

Articulating Forceps and Articulating Paper

Use	• To hold articulating paper when checking the patient's occlusion after the filling material has been placed • To mark patient's occlusion and check bite
Parts	Handle with long beaks that secure the articulating paper • Paper of various thickness, from ultra-thin to thick • Comes in rolls or individual strips
Misc.	• May be made of stainless steel; this type is opened and closed by placing pressure on the handle to allow for articulating paper to be inserted and removed. May also be made of disposable plastic; in this type the articulating paper is held in position by closing and securing the beaks. • Articulating paper comes in blue, red, black, and green. It is available on rolls, as individual strips, and in horseshoe shapes. • Articulating paper can be stored in easy-access dispensers. • Articulating paper is coated with liquid colors on both sides to facilitate accurate marking of occlusal contact and interferences.

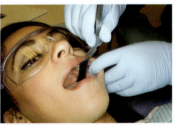

Copyright © 2015 Cengage Learning®.

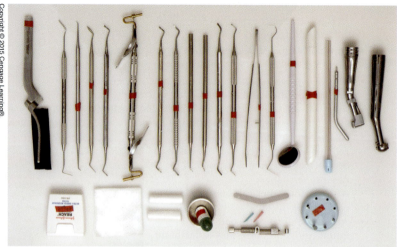

Amalgam Tray Setup

- Top of the tray: burs in bur block; matrix band, Tofflemire retainer, and wedges; amalgam well; amalgam capsules; cotton rolls; gauze sponges; floss
- Bottom of the tray: high- and low-speed handpieces, air-water syringe, saliva ejector, high-volume evacuator (HVE) tip, mouth mirror, explorer, cotton pliers, spoon excavator, hatchet, binangle chisel, hoe, mesial and distal gingival margin trimmers, amalgam carrier, amalgam condenser, Hollenback carver, cleoid-discoid carver, ICP carver, articulating paper forceps, and articulating paper
- Off-tray items include anesthetic, rubber dam, amalgamator, liners, and bases.

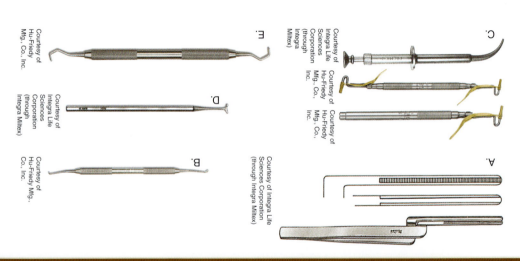

A.

Courtesy of Integra Life
Sciences Corporation
(through Integra Miltex)

B.

Courtesy of
Hu-Friedy Mfg.,
Co., Inc.

C.

Courtesy of
Integra Life
Sciences
Corporation
(through
Integra
Miltex)

Courtesy of
Hu-Friedy
Mfg.. Co.,
Inc.

Courtesy of
Hu-Friedy Mfg.. Co.,
Inc.

D.

Courtesy of
Integra Life
Sciences
Corporation
(through
Integra Miltex)

E.

Courtesy of
Hu-Friedy
Mfg.. Co.. Inc.

_____ 1. This instrument is used to place amalgam filling material into the cavity preparation.

_____ 2. This instrument has a disc on one end and a spade on the other.

_____ 3. This instrument is used to hold articulating paper.

_____ 4. This instrument allows the dentist to access difficult-to-reach areas when placing amalgam .

_____ 5. This instrument is used to smooth rough margins of restorations and to shape metal matrix bands.

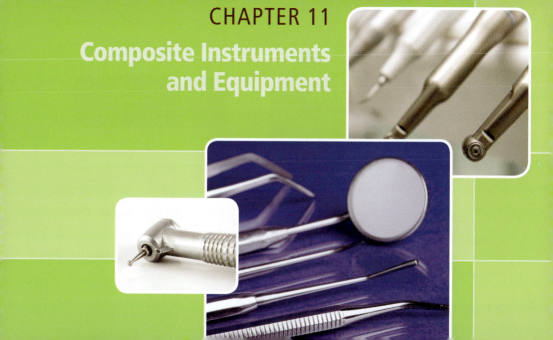

Composite Shade Guide

A.

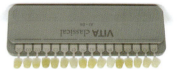

B.

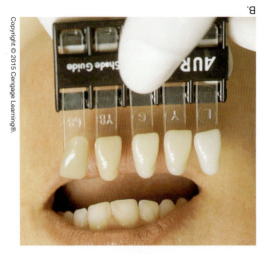

| Use | To obtain correct shade for composite restoration to match patient's current tooth shade (See other uses in Chapter 17, Fixed Prosthodontic Instruments.) |

Use

To obtain correct shade for composite restoration to match patient's current tooth shade (See other uses in Chapter 17, Fixed Prosthodontic Instruments.)

Parts

- A guide with multiple tooth shades on removable tabs that are labeled to indicate shade with letters and numbers

A. Vita shade guide shown
B. Obtaining a shade under natural light at the beginning of the procedure

Misc.

- A different shade may be used for the gingival third, the middle third, and/or the incisal third of the restoration.
- Many different shade guides are available.
- Digital or electric shade guides can select an overall single tooth shade or can select separate shades for the gingival, middle, and incisal thirds. The digital device can send the information on the shade to dental laboratories.
- Shade guides often come with the composite kits.

A.

B.

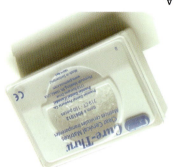

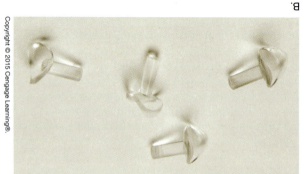

Use	To compress and contour restorative material into cervical area as it is light cured
Parts	**A.** A plastic tab attached to a contoured matrix that fits the cervical area of the tooth
	B. Some cervical matrices come with a positioning instrument instead of a tab.
Misc.	• Available in an assorted box of 250
	• Contains (50) anterior/premolar and molar matrices
	• Contains (35) matrices in other shapes
	• Comes with a positioning instrument, which is also clear
	• Flexible to fit the exact contour of the tooth
	• Allows for excellent marginal integrity
	• Material can be cured directly through this matrix
	• For composite interproximal matrix, a plastic strip matrix is used. See Chapter 9, Diagnostic Aids, Matrices, and Instruments for Cements, Bases, and Liners.

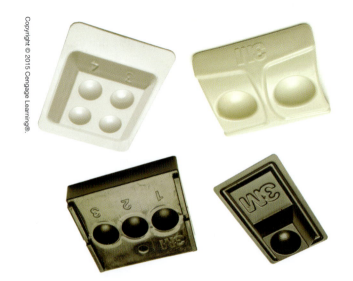

Well For Composite Material

Use	To hold material: etchant, bonding, or composite material
Parts	• Disposable or autoclavable holder with different wells • Many have orange covers to block the materials from light, which initiates setting.
Misc.	• Wells are labeled with numbers or letters to designate different materials. • Wells can be single, double, triple, or more. • Wells often come with the composite kits or material.

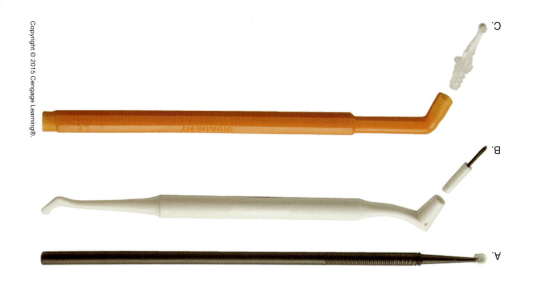

A.

B.

C.

Applicator

Use   To apply conditioner, primer, etchant, and bonding material to cavity preparation

Parts   **A.** One-piece applicator, available in many colors to note material being used, The working end bends.
B. Microbrush applicator, available in many sizes and styles
C. Two-piece applicator, available in autoclavable handle and removable tip

Misc.   • Disposable applicator or tip
• Comes in large quantity
• Several colors in each package

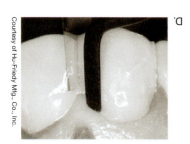

D.

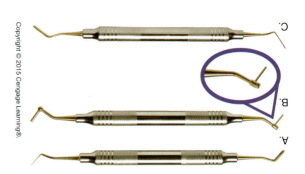

C.

B.

A.

Composite Placement Instrument

Use	• To carry composite material to and from cavity preparation
	• To place and condense composite material in the cavity preparation
	• To rough carve composite material after it has been placed in the cavity preparation
Parts	Double-ended instrument with different angles and working ends
	A. Placement and contouring instrument
	B. Condensing instrument
	C. Placement and contouring instrument
	D. The working end of a placement instrument on the tooth
Misc.	• Available in a variety of shapes, angles, and sizes
	• Available in metal or plastic
	• Each end of the instrument is used differently: one end is used to place the material; the other end is used to contour and rough carve the material.

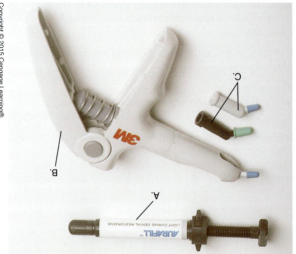

A.

B.

C.

Composite Syringes and Cartridges

Use

Packaged one-paste composite systems that come in a syringe or a single-dose cartridge that is used with a syringe to place the material in the cavity preparation or on the composite well/paper pad for delivery with the composite placement instrument

Parts

A. Composite one-paste syringe for several applications
B. Composite syringe
C. Single-dosage cartridges to be used with the composite syringe

Misc.

- Come in many shades
- Shade guides accompany each composite system.

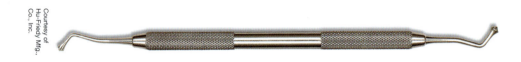

Composite Burnisher

Use	• To smooth, contour, and form occlusal anatomy in composite restorations
	• To attain the anatomical grooves, pits, and fissures
Parts	• Double-ended instrument
	• Different angle on each end of the instrument
	• The tip is often shaped like an acorn.
	A. Composite burnisher
	B. Contact former
Misc.	• The composite burnisher is available in titanium-nitride coating or gold-titanium-nitride coating, which resists scratching and discoloration of composite material. It allows for a smooth surface due to the nonstick surface of the tip of the instrument.

CHAPTER 11 Composite Instruments and Equipment

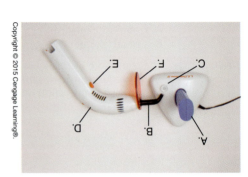

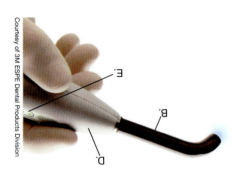

Curing Light

Use	Used to "cure" or "set" light-cured materials

Parts

A. Battery pack
B. Wands or tips
C. Radiometer
D. Motor
E. Triggers to activate the light
F. Protective shield

Misc.

- The curing light can be battery powered as shown or electric, where the light is attached to the motor with a cord.
- Some curing lights have digital display countdown timers and preset curing times.
- The dental materials that are to be cured must be cured in increments of 2 mm or less to ensure complete setting.
- A testing device (radiometer) or meter is used to evaluate the accuracy of the curing light (see G above).

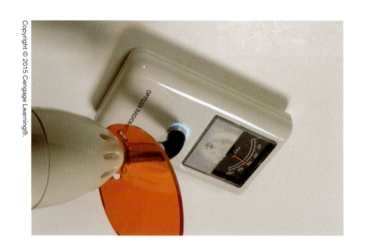

Curing Light Meter

Use	To test the curing lights to ensure that the correct level of power is emitted

Parts   Radiometer with area for curing light tip placement to check accuracy of the output; a gauge on the radiometer is present to show the reading.

Misc.
- Lights should be tested at least once a month.
- There are radiometers for both the halogen and light-emitting diode (LED) curing lights.
- If the material does not appear to be setting, the light should be tested immediately.
- The curing lights are continually improving, and newer devices are available for testing.

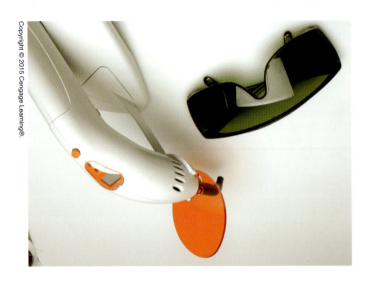

Protective Shield for Curing Light

Use	To protect the operator and auxiliary's eyes during the curing of dental materials
Parts	• Glasses can be used with orange- or green-colored lenses. • Handheld or paddle devices of green- or orange-colored shields can be used. • Shields are attached to most curing lights.
Misc.	• Many of the curing units have protective orange shields available. • Most curing lights come with a shield attached. • The shields can be disinfected.

Composite Polishers

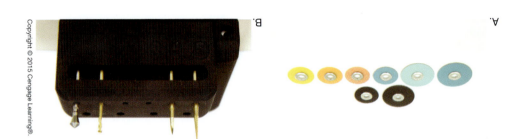

A.

B.

To contour, refine, and polish the composite restorative material

Parts
- Metal-centered disc that adapts to the mandrel
- Synthetic material impregnated with types of grit
- Synthetic material snap-on discs of various grits, shown by different colors

A. Centerless composite discs to be used on mandrels
B. Composite polishers on mandrels in various shapes

Misc.
- Available in a range of grits, from extra-fine to coarse
- Often color coded according to grit
- Available in a variety of shapes and sizes
- The discs are disposable; some come with disposable mandrels.
- The darker the color of the disc, the more abrasive it is.

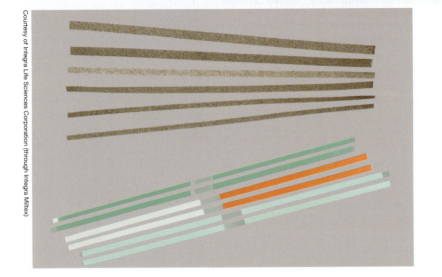

Finishing Strip

Use	To smooth and finish the interproximal surfaces of composite restorations
Parts	Strips of synthetic fabric that are abrasive to remove excess restorative material from the interproximal area
Misc.	• Available in different grit consistencies • Many have no abrasive material in the center of the strip. This allows the operator to slide the strip between the teeth without removing tooth structure and/or the proximal of the restoration.

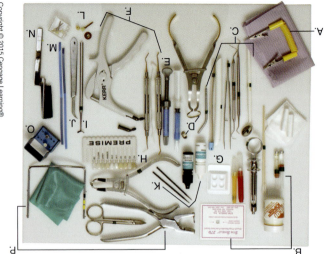

Composite Procedure Tray

Use	To assist in the preparation of cavity preparation and placement and the finishing of a composite restoration
Parts	**A.** Bib and clip
	B. Anesthetic: topical applicators, carpules, needle shield, syringe, needle
	C. Basic setup: mirror, explorer, cotton, forceps (pliers), air-water syringe (three-way syringe), high-velocity (volume) evacuation (HVE) tip, saliva ejector, and spoon excavator
	D. Matrices with placement forceps
	E. Etchant
	F. Composite placement instruments and composite material
	G. Composite well
	H. Shade guide
	I. Composite burnisher
	J. #12 blade and scalpel
	K. Etchant applicator tips, bonding applicator tips, and primer
	L. Composite finishing discs
	M. Composite finishing strip
	N. Articulating paper and holder
	O. Burs and bur holder (handpieces not shown)
	P. Dental dam setup

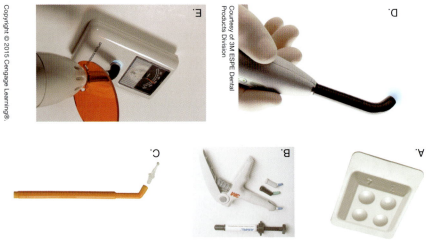

Test Your Knowledge

A.

B.

C.

D.

Courtesy of 3M ESPE Dental Products Division

E.

_____ 1. Identify the instrument that is used to apply the conditioner, primer, and bonding material to the cavity preparation.

_____ 2. Identify the well for the composite material.

_____ 3. Identify the instrument that is the composite syringe and cartridge.

_____ 4. Identify the item that ensures that the correct level of power is emitted from the curing light.

_____ 5. Identify the item that sets the dental material.

Endodontic Instruments

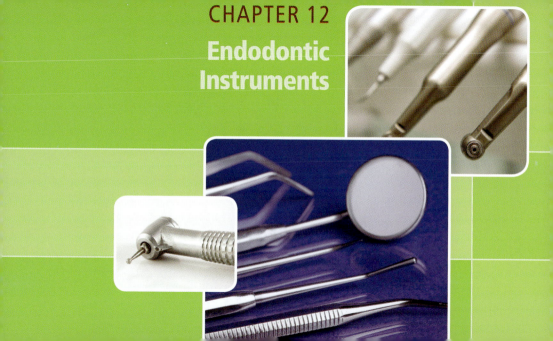

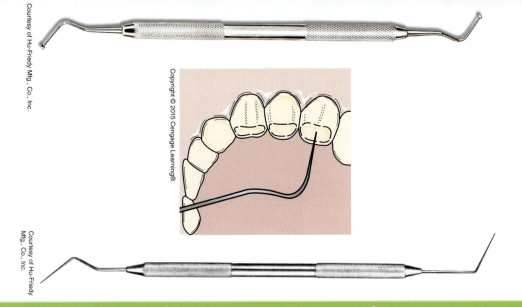

Endodontic Explorer and Endodontic Spoon Excavator

Use	• The explorer is used to assist in locating canal (orifices) openings.
	• The spoon excavator is used to reach into the coronal portion of the tooth; to reach the bottom of the pulp chamber; and to remove deep caries, pulp tissue, and temporary cement.
Parts	• The explorer has long tapered ends that have sharp points.
	• The spoon excavator has a very long shank to reach into the pulp chamber.
	• The instruments are double ended.
Misc.	• The explorer's long tapered ends allow for exploration and finding the canals.
	• The stiff-ended explorer is designed specifically for endodontic procedures.
	• Available in a variety of sizes

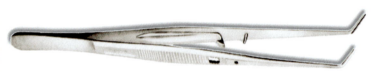

Endodontic Locking Pliers

| **Use** | To grasp and transport various materials to and from the oral cavity |

Parts
- Locking handles to secure items for transfer, placement, and retrieval
- Similar to tweezers, with smooth surfaces or serrations on the ends of the beaks

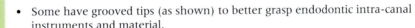

Misc.
- Some have grooved tips (as shown) to better grasp endodontic intra-canal instruments and material.

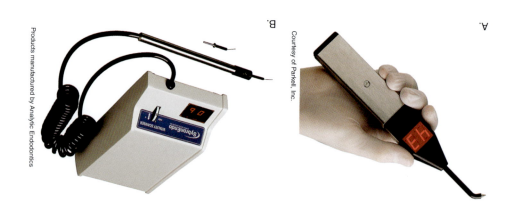

Pulp Tester and Vitality Scanner

A.

Courtesy of Parkell, Inc.

B.

Products manufactured by Analytic Endodontics

Use	To test each tooth for vitality
Parts	

- Vitality scanner unit includes
  - Long probe tip
  - Short probe tip
  - Mini probe tip
  - Lip clip
  - Grounding lead with lip clip
- There are two types:
  - **A.** Battery operated
  - **B.** Electronic with digital display

Misc.

- They deliver high-frequency stimuli to the tooth, which causes a reaction if the tooth is vital.
- The impulse is slowly increased until the patient indicates sensitivity.
- With some units, toothpaste is applied to the coronal surface of the tooth where the probe tip is placed. The toothpaste acts as a conductor.
- Some units give readouts on the vitality of the tooth.

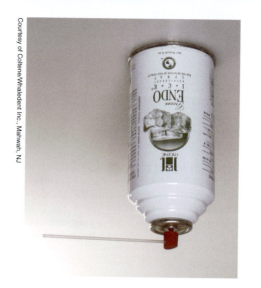

Endo Ice

| **Use** | • To check the sensitivity of the tooth |
| | • To check the vitality of the tooth |

Parts Dry ice, ethyl chloride, or a piece of ice

Misc.
- Many brands available
- Some are much cooler than ice or ethyl chloride.
- Do not require refrigeration

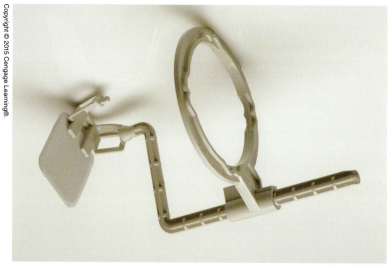

Endodontic X-Ray Film Holder

Use	Film holder designed specifically for endodontic radiographs
Parts	Rod with a ring specially designed to hold the radiograph and obtain a quality x-ray of an endodontic tooth showing the apex
Misc.	

- The film holder can be used to expose radiographs on the maxillary and mandibular teeth on both the anterior and posterior areas.
- The endodontic film holder allows for an x-ray to be exposed with a reamer in place.
- Designed to fit over rubber dam clamps and endodontic files
- The x-ray holder is used to take endodontic measurements.
- Available for digital or manual

Broaches

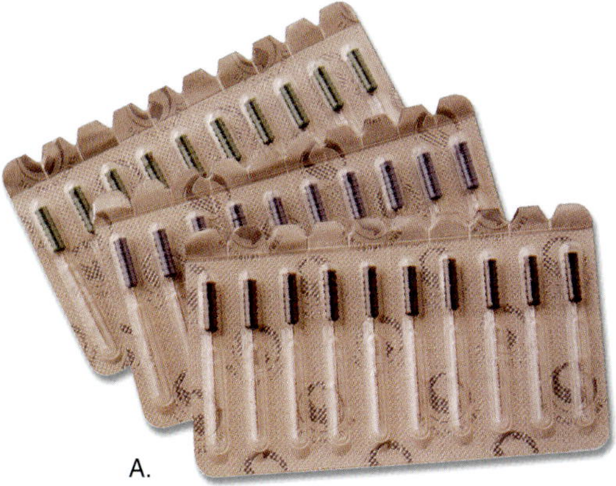

A.

Courtesy of Sybron Endo (Orange, CA)

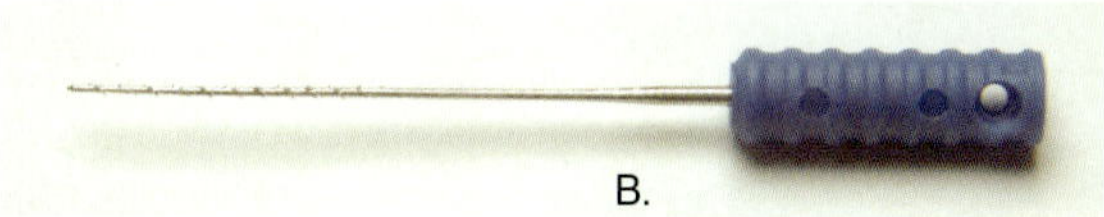

B.

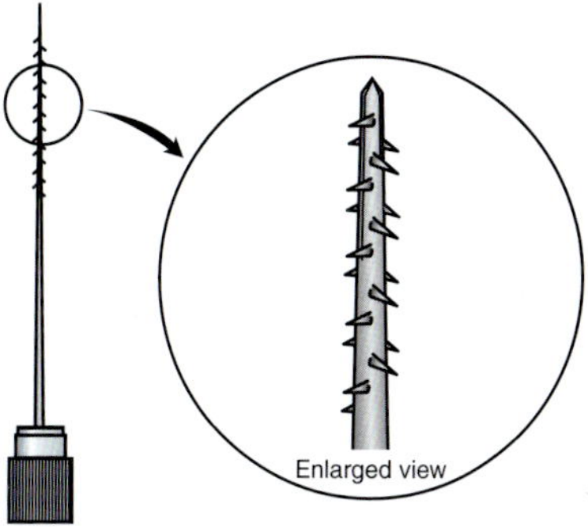

C.

Enlarged view

Use

To remove soft tissue from the pulp canal (extirpate)

Parts

- Fine metal wire with tiny, sharp projections or barbs along the instrument shaft

  A. Packages of barbed broaches in various diameters
  B. Single barbed broach
  C. Close-up drawing of a barbed broach

Misc.

- Broaches come in individual sterile cell packs.
- Broaches are discarded after one use.
- Barbed broaches are supplied in various diameters, ranging from xxxx-fine to coarse.
- Color-coded plastic handles make proper size selection easier.
- Also comes with a notched end to be used with an endodontic handpiece

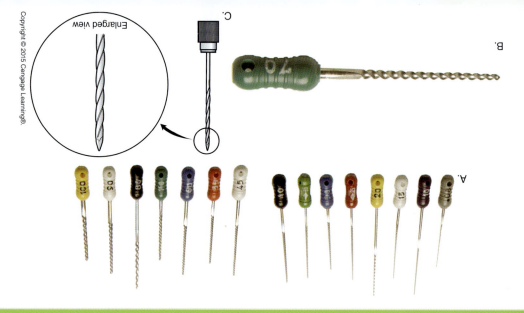

K-Type Files

A.

B.

C.

Enlarged view

| **Use** | • To scrape and widen the walls of the canal |
| | • To remove necrotic tissue |

Use
- To scrape and widen the walls of the canal
- To remove necrotic tissue

Parts
- Stainless steel with a tightly twisted design
- Handles are color coded according to size

    A. Variety of K-type files
    B. Single K-type file
    C. Close-up of tip of the K-type file

Misc.
- K-type files are twisted into the canal.
- Also available in nickel-titanium for more flexibility
- Also comes with a notched end to be used with an endodontic handpiece
- Available in various diameters to match the width of the canals
- Available in different lengths, for example: 21 mm, 25 mm, 28 mm, and 31 mm

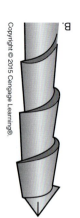

B.

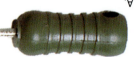

A.

Hedstrom Files

Use	• To scrape and widen the walls of the canal
	• To remove necrotic tissue
	• To smooth the walls of the canal

Use
- To scrape and widen the walls of the canal
- To remove necrotic tissue
- To smooth the walls of the canal

Parts
- The edges are very sharp and cut aggressively.
- The handles are color coded according to size.
- Also comes with a notched end to be used with an endodontic handpiece

  A. Hedstrom file
  B. Close-up of the tip of a Hedstrom file

Misc.
- These files are used only in a push-and-pull motion so they will not bind in the canal.
- Manufactured by a different process
- They are shaped like pine trees and appear to look like a stack of cones.
- Available in various diameters to match the width of the canals
- Available in different lengths, for example: 21 mm, 25 mm, 28 mm, and 31 mm

Courtesy of Sybron Dental

Use	• For curved and narrow canals
	• To scrape and widen the walls of the canal
	• To remove necrotic tissue
Parts	• Made of stainless steel or nickel-titanium
	• Handles are color coded according to size.
	• Also comes with a notched end to be used with an endodontic handpiece
Misc.	• Crafted for optimal balance of flexibility, strength, and sharpness
	• Available in various diameters to match the width of the canals
	• Different lengths, for example: 21 mm and 25 mm

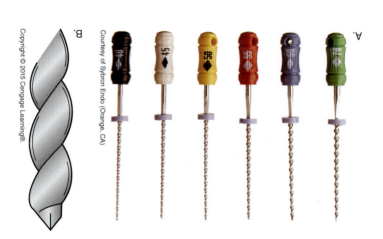

Reamer

A.

Courtesy of Sybron Endo (Orange, CA)

B.

Copyright © 2015 Cengage Learning®.

Use

- To clean and enlarge the canal walls
- To smooth the walls of the canal

Parts

- Have twisted shanks like the files, but the blades are spaced much farther apart
- The handles are color coded and numbered according to size, similar to the files.
- Also comes with a notched end to be used with an endodontic handpiece

    A. Selection of reamers in various diameters
    B. Close-up view showing spiral cutting edges

Misc.

- Reamers are used with a "reaming" or twisting motion.
- Similar to a K-type file, but has fewer twists; therefore the cutting edges are further apart.
- Available in different lengths, for example: 21 mm, 25 mm, 28 mm, and 31 mm

Endo Organizers and Endodontic Measuring Device/Millimeter Ruler

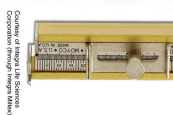

C.

A.

B.

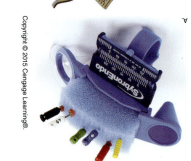

Use	• To store and organize reamers and files
	• To measure length of endodontic reamer or file and mark with rubber stoppers
Parts	• Measurement device with area to hold endodontic broaches, reamers, or files

A. Ring plastic with disposable sponge endodontic organizer

B. Stainless steel endodontic organizer with ruler

C. Millimeter rulers with a finger clip or attached to an endodontic organizer

The ruler has an adjustable indicator that shows the length of the stop position

Misc.	• Some of the storage containers can be sterilized.
	• Some are designed to hold a range of intracanal instruments.
	• Large organizers often have measuring gauges for setting stops.
	• Finger rings are much smaller, holding only a few instruments at once.
	• Available in stainless steel or plastic
	• Some of the units can be sterilized.
	• The smaller handheld units often have disposable sponges.

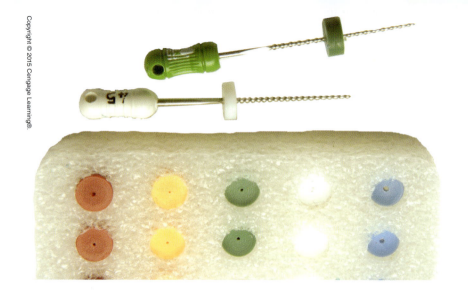

Endodontic Measuring Stops

Use	To place on reamers and files to mark the length of the root canal
Parts	Small, circular, silicone disks of various colors
Misc.	

- Endodontic measuring stops are also known as rubber stops or markers.
- The length of the canal is determined by holding a file with a rubber stop against a radiograph and adjusting the stop to match the incisal or cusp edge.
- The marked file is then measured on a small millimeter gauge.
- This number is recorded for reference and for marking other intracanal instruments.

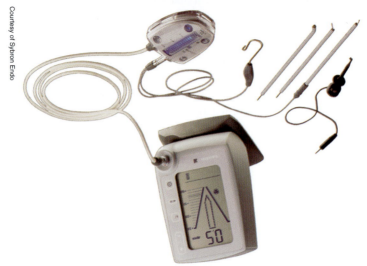

Apex Locator

Use	To locate the apex of the tooth and display the information on a digital readout
Parts	An electronic unit with display screen that shows the length of the apex through multiple-frequency technology
Misc.	• Many units have visual readouts and audible alerts. • Attaches to reamer or file and placed in canal • It can work in either wet or dry environments.

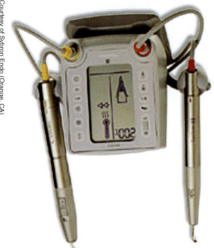

Courtesy of Sybron Endo (Orange, CA)

Gutta Percha Obturation System

Use	• To soften the gutta percha before placing it in the canal
	• To backfill, cauterize, and hot pulp test
Parts	A unit with control console with a digital display, an extruder handpiece, and a second handpiece used for downfilling, backfilling, cauterizing, and hot pulp testing; has a temperature control
Misc.	• Temperature can be controlled to adjust the viscosity of the gutta percha.
	• Many types are available, with various function combinations.

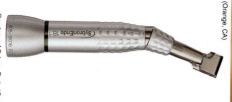

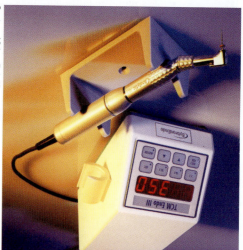

Endodontic Handpiece

Use	• To mechanically clean and enlarge the root canal
	• To place the endodontic sealer in the canal

Use
- To mechanically clean and enlarge the root canal
- To place the endodontic sealer in the canal

Parts
- A slow-speed electric torque motor with foot control with display controls to set speed and torque level
- Area for endodontic attachments

Misc.
- Attaches to a slow-speed handpiece
- Consistently and evenly supplies quarter-turn motion
- Used with reamers, files, and Lentulo spirals during endodontic procedures

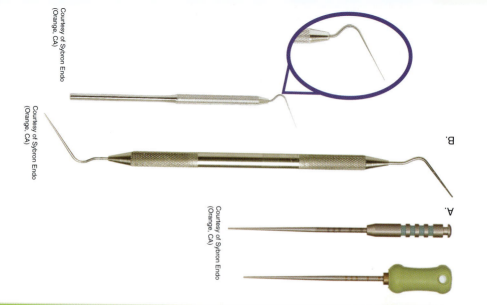

B.

A.

Endodontic Spreaders

| **Use** | • To laterally condense materials when obturating (sealing/filling) the canal |
| | • To adapt the gutta percha (root canal filling material) into the canal |

Parts
- Spreaders are pointed on the ends.

  A. Finger spreaders, hand and slow-speed attached spreaders
  B. Double- and single-ended hand spreaders

Misc.
- Some spreaders have short handles that are rotated and held by the fingers; thus they are called "finger spreaders."
- Single or double ended
- Sized to correspond to canal size
- Rings in millimeter increments are found on the working end.

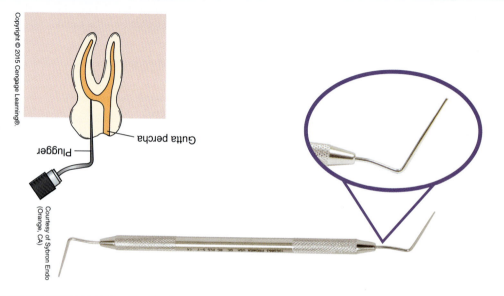

Gutta percha

Plugger

Courtesy of Sybron Endo (Orange, CA)

Endodontic Pluggers

Use	To vertically condense material when obturating (sealing/filling) the canal
Parts	• Single ended
	• Flat ends
	• Short and long handles
Misc.	• Available in various sizes to fit into the canals

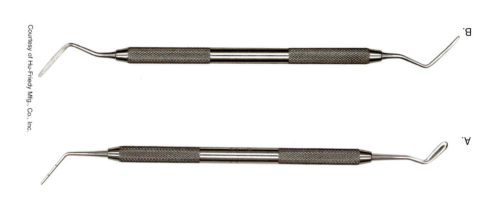

B.

A.

Glick Endodontic Instruments

Use	• To remove excess gutta percha from the coronal portion of the canal
	• To condense the remaining gutta percha in the canal opening
	• To carry and place gutta percha

Use
- To remove excess gutta percha from the coronal portion of the canal
- To condense the remaining gutta percha in the canal opening
- To carry and place gutta percha

Parts
- Long, tapered spoon on each end
- Doubled ended

    A. #1 Glick
    B. #2 Glick

Misc.
- May have millimeter rings on plugger end
- Available in a variety of working ends

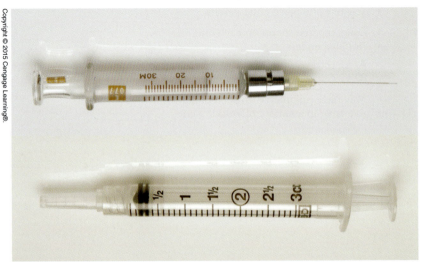

Endodontic Irrigation Syringe/Luer Lock Syringe

Use	• To irrigate the canal during and after use of the files and reamers • To debride (cleanse) the canal
Parts	• Calibrated barrel: comes in different sizes, for example 3 cc or 12 cc • Plunger • Needle: 23, 27, or 30 gauge
Misc.	• Plastic: disposable • Glass: nonsterile with disposable tips

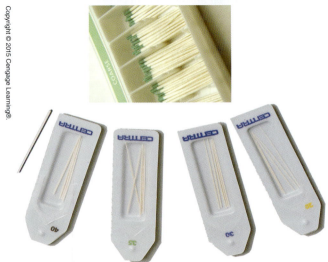

Absorbent Paper Points

- To dry canals (placed in the canal until canal is dry)
- To place medications in the canal
- To take cultures of the canal

Parts   Paper points are absorbent and in the shape of a long narrow cone.

Misc.

- Supplied in various sizes, from x-fine to coarse
- Available in sterile and nonsterile
- Some are color coded to match the endodontic files.
- The sizes match the length and width of the canal.
- Several points are used to ensure the canal is dry.

A.

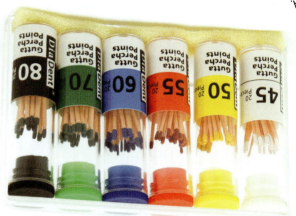

B.

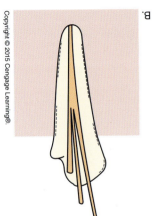

	To obdurate (fill) the root canal after the canal has been opened and cleaned
Use	

Parts	• Thermoplastic material that is flexible at room temperature yet stiff enough to be placed in the root canal
	• Comes in cones that are supplied in graduated sizes, from x-fine to large
	• The gutta percha and cores are heated with special heating units before being inserted into the canal.
	
	   A. Various gutta percha kits
	   B. Gutta percha shown in root canal prior to removing ends in crown of tooth

Misc.	• Some are color coded to match endodontic files. • Some are radiopaque so they can be seen on radiographs. • Thermal gutta percha endodontic obturation systems are also available; these systems include metal cores coated with gutta percha.

Gates-Glidden Drills

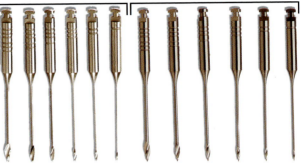

A.

Courtesy of Integra Life Sciences Corporation (through Integra Miltex)

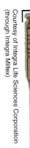

B.

Courtesy of Sybron Endo (Orange, CA)

| **Use** | • To prepare the opening access in the coronal portion of the canal |
| | • To widen the upper portion of the canal for better access |

| **Parts** | Long shanked bur with various-sized cutting ends |

A. Various-sized Gates-Glidden drills
B. Line art showing Gates-Glidden drill in canal of tooth

Misc.	• Latch-type bur used with contra-angle low-speed handpiece
	• Elliptical (football-shaped) cutting ends
	• Supplied in six sizes, marked by the number of grooves on the shank
	• Sizes are compatible with all endodontic instruments.
	• Two lengths: longer for anterior teeth and shorter for posterior teeth

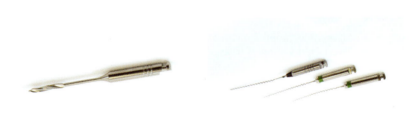

Lentulo Spiral and Peeso Reamer

Use	• The Lentulo spiral is used to place and evenly distribute root canal sealer or cement in the canal.
	• The Peeso reamer is used to prepare the canal for a post and to reduce the curvature for the canal orifice for straight-line access.
Parts	• The Lentulo spiral is a long, twisted, very flexible wire instrument.
	• The Peeso reamer is a latch type; it is used with a contra-angle attachment on a low-speed handpiece and has parallel cutting sides.
Misc.	• Spirals are used with low-speed handpieces and contra-angle attachments.
	• If a Lentulo spiral becomes bent it should not be reused.
	• The Lentulo spiral attachment end is latched.
	• The Peeso reamer is supplied in various sizes; the shanks are marked with grooves to indicate the corresponding size.

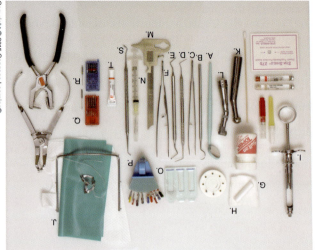

Root Canal Therapy—Opening Appointment Tray Setup

A. Mouth mirror
B. Explorer
C. Cotton pliers
D. Endodontic explorer
E. Endodontic spoon excavator
F. Locking cotton pliers
G. Cotton rolls
H. Gauze sponges
I. Anesthetic setup
J. Dental dam setup
K. High-speed handpiece
L. Low-speed handpiece
M. Millimeter ruler
N. Irrigating syringe and solution
O. Paper points
P. Barbed broach, assorted reamers and files with stops in endodontic organizer
Q. Peeso reamers
R. Gates-Glidden drills
S. Glick endodontic instrument
T. Temporary filling material

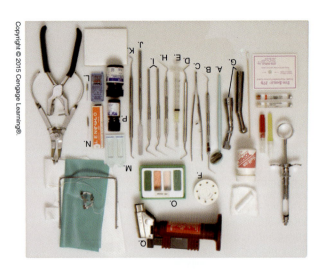

Root Canal Therapy–Closing Appointment Tray Setup

A. Mouth mirror
B. Endodontic explorer
C. Locking cotton pliers
D. Endodontic spoon excavator
E. Irrigating syringe
F. Burs
G. High- and low-speed handpieces
H. Spreaders
I. Pluggers
J. Spatula
K. Glick instrument
L. Gates-Glidden drills
M. Absorbent sterile paper points
N. Lentulo spiral
O. Gutta percha
P. Root canal sealer
Q. Heat source

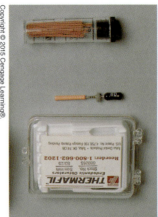

Thermal Obturation System

Use

Parts

To place the gutta percha into the canal

- Plastic- or metal-core gutta percha obturators

  A. Heating unit with obturators
  B. Close-up of obturator with and without gutta percha

Misc.

- The gutta percha obturators are heated in the heating units and then inserted into the canal.
- The handle of the obturator is then removed with a bur.

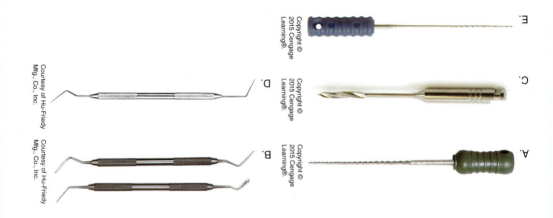

E.

Copyright © 2015 Cengage Learning®.

C.

Copyright © 2015 Cengage Learning®.

A.

Copyright © 2015 Cengage Learning®.

D.

Courtesy of Hu-Friedy Mfg., Co., Inc.

B.

Courtesy of Hu-Friedy Mfg., Co., Inc.

_____ 1. Identify the Glick endodontic instrument.

_____ 2. Identify the endodontic instrument that is used to locate the canal openings.

_____ 3. Identify the instrument that is used at the beginning of the procedure to remove soft tissue from the pulp canal.

_____ 4. Identify the Hedstrom file.

_____ 5. Identify the instrument used to place cement in the root canal.

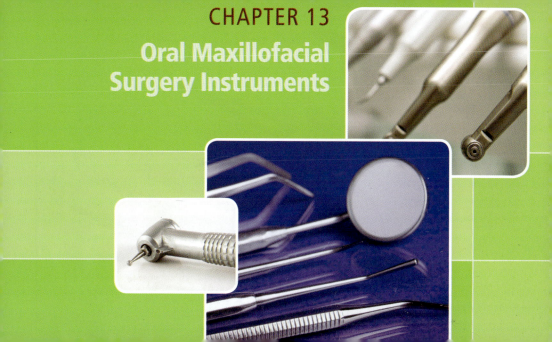

CHAPTER 13

Oral Maxillofacial Surgery Instruments

A. holds scalpel blade

B. incise or excise soft tissue

#11

#12

#15

C.

Use	To precisely incise or excise soft tissue with the least amount of trauma

Parts

A. Handles: These are slim and straight and are designed to accommodate detachable disposable blades. Handles are flat and often have a metric ruler on them.

B. Disposable blades (scalpel): These come in various shapes and sizes and are very sharp. They are supplied in sterile packages and disposed of after one use. Common blades are:
- #15 for surgical procedures
- #11 to incise and drain
- #13 to incise and drain

C. Disposable scalpels are also available. These have plastic handles with metal blades and are supplied in sterile packages and disposed of after one use.

Misc.

- They are made from stainless steel or are disposable.
- Scalpel and blades are used in surgery and periodontal surgical procedures as well as in finishing composite restorations.

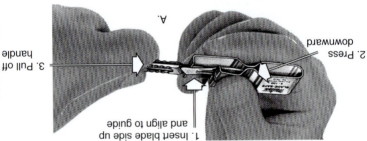

A.

1. Insert blade side up and align to guide

2. Press downward

3. Pull off handle

B.

Hu-Friedy
SCALPEL BLADE
REMOVER
Stainless/Germany
Pat. Pend.

PRESS
10-199-00

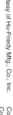

Courtesy of Hu-Friedy Mfg., Co., Inc.

Courtesy of Integra Life Sciences Corporation (through Integra Miltex)

| **Use** | To remove the blades from the blade handle |
| **Parts** | • Slotted metal device to allow the blade to fit into it for safety |

A. Blade being placed in remover
B. Scalpel blade remover

Misc.	• Application is to place the blade into the remover and to align with the notch
	• Press down on the blade remover.
	• Slowly pull away the handle from the blade, and the blade should remain within the remover.
	• Discard the blade in sharps container.

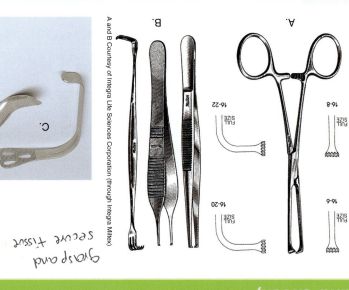

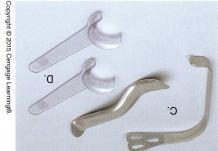

A.

16-8
FULL SIZE

16-6
FULL SIZE

16-22
FULL SIZE

16-20
FULL SIZE

B.

A and B Courtesy of Integra Life Sciences Corporation (through Integra Miltex)

C.

D.

grasp and
secure tissue

Tissue Forceps and Retractors (Lip, Tongue, and Cheek)

Use

- To hold tissue from the surgical site so that the view of the operator is unobstructed
- To hold the lip, tongue, and cheeks out of the way so the operator can view the site during the procedure

Parts

Tissue Forceps:

A. Forceps (hinged types)
B. Cotton-plier style and straight hand grasp instrument

- The working end of both types has small teeth to assist in securely grasping the tissue.

Lip, Tongue, and Cheek Retractors:

C. Spoon or blade shaped at different angles for tongue and oral cavity
D. Arch shaped for cheeks and lips

- Placed on the buccal mucosa, and then the tissue is retracted for a clear view

Misc.

- Available in a variety of shapes and styles

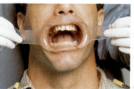

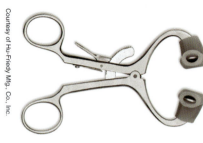

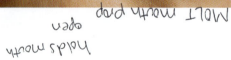

Molt mouth prop

holds mouth open

Mouth Gag

| **Use** | To prevent the patient's mouth from closing during the procedure |

Parts
- Hinged device with ratchet release
- Handles and beaks

Misc.
- The application is to close the beaks and insert into the patient's mouth.
- The handle is gently squeezed, which opens the beaks and the patient's mouth.
- The forceps are locked in this position until the release is engaged.
- Supplied in pediatric, child, and adult sizes

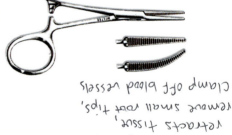

Courtesy of Integra Life Sciences Corporation (through Integra Miltex)

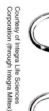
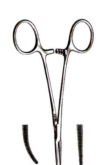

(A) Courtesy of Integra Life Sciences Corporation (through Integra Miltex) (B) Courtesy of Hu-Friedy Mfg., Co., Inc.

Grab loose objects,
retracts tissue,
remove small vent tips,
clamp off blood vessels

holds needle of suture

Hemostats and Needle Holders

Use	• To retract tissue

<table>
<tr><td>Use</td><td><ul><li>To retract tissue</li><li>To remove small root tips</li><li>To clamp off blood vessels</li><li>To grasp loose objects</li><li>To grasp and handle suture needle during suturing procedure</li></ul></td></tr>
<tr><td>Parts</td><td><ul><li>Working ends that are long, serrated, or grooved beaks</li><li>Locking handles can be manipulated with one hand.</li><li>The beaks of the needle holder are shorter than those of the hemostat.</li><li>The needle holder has fine serrations with a groove down the center of each beak to hold the suture needle.</li></ul></td></tr>
<tr><td>Misc.</td><td><ul><li>Various sizes</li><li>Various types, including Kelly and the Halstead-Mosquito</li><li>Available with straight or curved beaks</li></ul></td></tr>
</table>

Suture or close
surgical sites

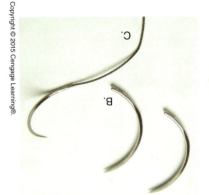

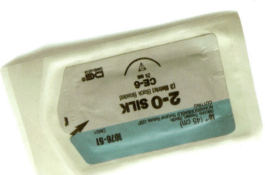

A.

B.

C.

2-0 SILK
NONABSORBABLE Surgical Suture USP
CUTTING
(3 Metric) Black Braided
CE-6
24 mm

18" (45 cm)

1076-51

Use	To suture (or close up with thread) the surgical site

Parts

A. Available in sterile package with suture attached to needle
B. Suture needle
C. Suture needle with suture attached

Misc.

- Available in a variety of suture needle sizes and different suture material
- Resorbable sutures: chromic gut, gut plain, and polyglycolic
- Available in sterile packets
- Non-resorbable sutures: nylon, polyester, polypropylene, and silk (most popular)

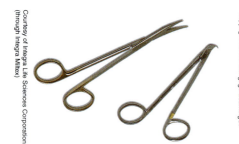

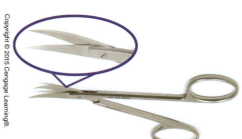

Cut sutures and trim soft tissue

Suture Scissors and Surgical Scissors

Use	• To cut sutures
	• To trim soft tissue
Parts	• Stainless steel
	• Suture scissors have a C-shaped notched area to slide under the suture and allow for cutting to occur.
	• Surgical scissors have pointed beaks with straight or angled blades.
Misc.	• Supplied in various sizes and shapes
	• Often one side of the cutting blades has a serrated area that holds the tissue while cutting.

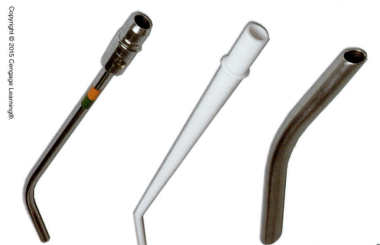

suction blood and debris
from surgical site

Surgical Aspirating Tips

Use	To aspirate blood and debris from the surgical site and back of the oral cavity for sedated patients
Parts	Long tubes that are very slender or tapered to small openings that attach to the high-volume suction
Misc.	• Made of plastic (disposable) or metal (sterilizable)

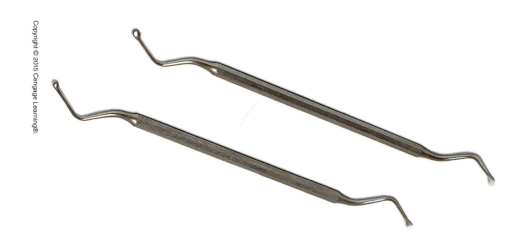

removes necrotic tissue

Surgical Curettes

Use	For curettage and debridement of the tooth socket or diseased tissue
Parts	• Double ended and have straight or curved shanks • The working end of the instrument is spoon shaped.
Misc.	• Available in various sizes

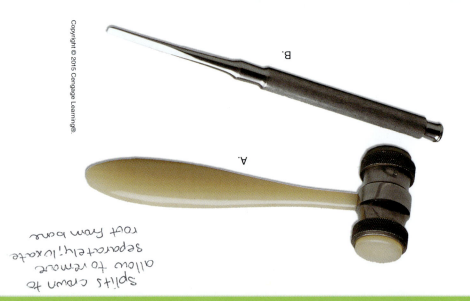

A.

B.

Splits crown to
allow to remove
separately; luxate
root from bone

Use	• The surgical mallet is used with the chisel to gently tap the end of the chisel. Together, they are used to split a tooth prior to removal.
	• Surgical chisels are used to remove or shape bone.
Parts	**A.** Surgical mallet
	B. Surgical chisel
Misc.	• Surgical chisels are available in beveled on one surface or bi-beveled on both sides.
	• Bi-beveled chisels are used for splitting a tooth.
	• Single-beveled chisels are used to remove and shape the bone.

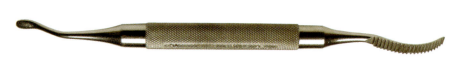

File, smooth, trim bone fragments

Surgical Bone File

Use	• To trim and smooth the bone after the teeth have been extracted
	• Used in a back-and-forth motion
Parts	• Usually double-ended instruments
	• The working end is normally rounded with serrations.
Misc.	• Available in various sizes and shapes

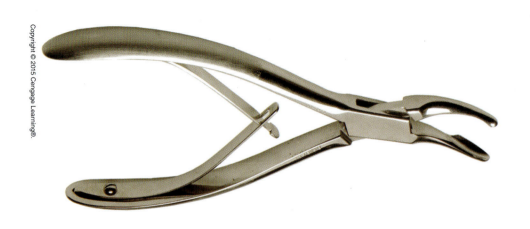

trim and shape alveolar bone

Rongeur (RON-jeer)

Use	To trim and shape the alveolar bone after extractions
Parts	• Hinged forceps with springs in the handle
	• Beaks are sharp and have cutting edges.
Misc.	• Available in different sizes and shapes

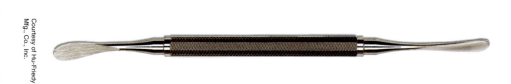

elevates periosteum and saliva

Periosteal Elevator

Use	
	• Has many uses and is included on most surgical tray setups
	• Often used to detach the periosteum (bone covering) and gingival tissues from around the tooth prior to the use of the extraction forceps
	• Also used to reflect and lift the mucoperiosteum (mucosa and periosteum) from the bone
Parts	
	• Double-ended instrument
	• Various working-end combinations
Misc.	
	• Often one end is pointed and the other end is rounded.
	• Available in various sizes and shapes

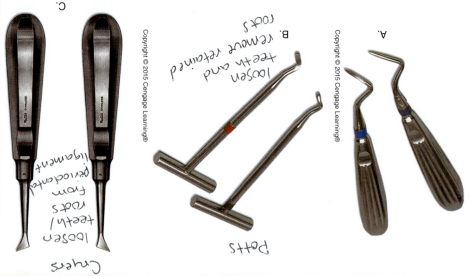

Elevators

A.

Copyright © 2015 Cengage Learning®

B. loosen teeth and remove retained roots

Potts

Copyright © 2015 Cengage Learning®

C.

loosen teeth/ roots from periodontal ligament

Cryers

(C) Courtesy of Integra Life Sciences Corporation (through Integra Miltex)

Use	To loosen and remove teeth, retained roots, and root fragments
Parts	<ul><li>Single-ended instruments with large bulbous or t-shaped handles to allow for a firm grip</li><li>The working ends of elevators may be straight or angular and are often paired left and right.</li><li>Common designer elevators are:</li></ul>

A. Apical—root tip
B. Potts—T-bar
C. Cryers—root

Misc.	<ul><li>Designed in different shapes and sizes</li></ul>

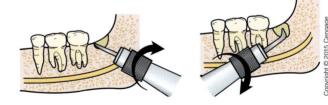

Copyright © 2015 Cengage Learning®.

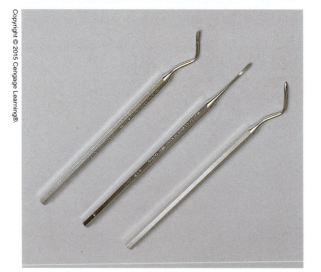

remove small retained root tips

Root Tip Picks

Use To elevate and remove root tips and fragments

Parts Slender instruments that have an elongated pointed working end.

Misc.
- They have either a slender or enlarged handle.
- Available in single or double ended
- Root tip picks are even thinner and longer than apical elevators.
- Root tip picks are paired left and right and are straight or angled.

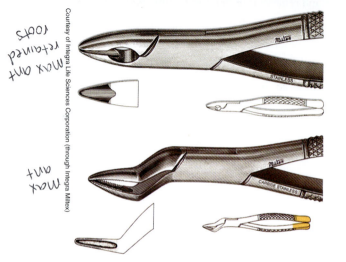

Max ant retained roots

Max ant

Extraction Forceps and #99C Maxillary Extraction Forceps

Use

To remove maxillary incisors and cuspids from the alveolar bone

Parts

- Handle
- Hinge
- Beak

Misc.

- Maxillary extraction forceps for incisors and root tips are commonly called bird-beak forceps.
- Hinged instruments with various handles and beak styles
- Specific forceps are used on certain teeth or in certain areas of the mouth.
- Each instrument has a number imprinted on the handle and is labeled with an "L" for left or "R" for right.
- Other forceps are designed according to the tooth morphology.

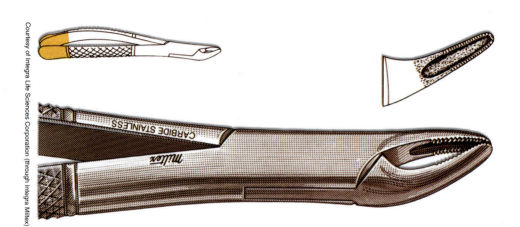

CARBIDE STAINLESS

miltex

max incisors, cuspids, bicuspids, retained roots

#150 Maxillary Extraction Forceps

Use	• Termed "universal forceps"
	• To remove maxillary incisors, cuspids, bicuspids, and roots
Parts	• Handle
	• Hinge
	• Beak
Misc.	• Hinged instruments with various handles and beak styles
	• Specific forceps are used on certain teeth or in certain areas of the mouth.
	• Each instrument has a number imprinted on the handle and is labeled with an "L" for left or "R" for right.
	• Other forceps are designed according to the tooth morphology.

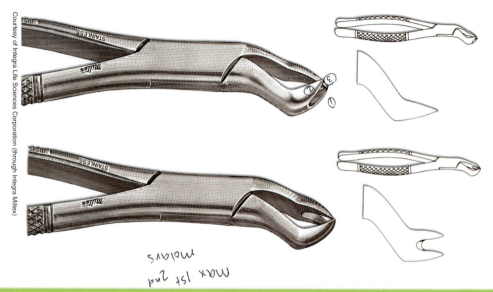

Max 1st 2nd
molars

Use

To remove first and second maxillary molars

Parts

- Handle
- Hinge
- Beak

Misc.

- Hinged instruments with various handles and beak styles
- Specific forceps are used on certain teeth or in certain areas of the mouth.
- Each instrument has a number imprinted on the handle and is labeled with an "L" for left or "R" for right.
- These forceps are designed according to the tooth morphology; the two beaked sides of the forceps are used to surround the lingual root, and one single side is used to go between the buccal roots in the bifurcation.

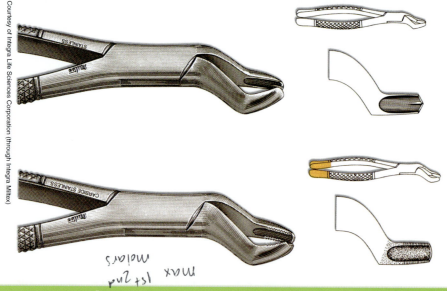

Max 1st 2nd molars

#53R and #53L Maxillary Extraction Forceps

Use	To remove maxillary first and second molars
Parts	<ul><li>Handle</li><li>Hinge</li><li>Beak</li></ul>
Misc.	<ul><li>Hinged instruments with various handles and beak styles</li><li>Specific forceps are used on certain teeth or in certain areas of the mouth.</li><li>Each instrument has a number imprinted on the handle and is labeled with an "L" for left or "R" for right.</li><li>Other forceps are designed according to the tooth morphology.</li></ul>

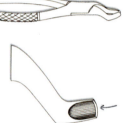

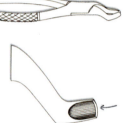

Courtesy of Integra Life Sciences Corporation
(through Integra Miltex)

Max 3rd
molars

#210 Maxillary Extraction Forceps

Use	• Termed "universal"
	• Used to remove maxillary third molars
Parts	• Handle
	• Hinge
	• Beak
Misc.	• Hinged instruments with various handles and beak styles
	• Specific forceps are used on certain teeth or in certain areas of the mouth.
	• Each instrument has a number imprinted on the handle and is labeled with an "L" for left or "R" for right.
	• Other forceps are designed according to the tooth morphology.

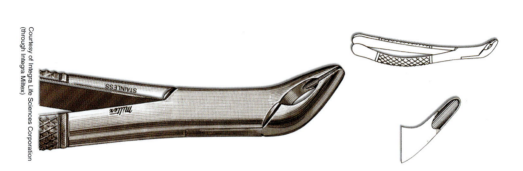

Man. incisors, cuspids, bicuspids, and roots

#203 Mandibular Extraction Forceps

Use	To remove mandibular incisors, biscuspids, cuspids, and roots
Parts	• Handle • Hinge • Beak
Misc.	• Hinged instruments with various handles and beak styles • Specific forceps are used on certain teeth or in certain areas of the mouth. • Each instrument has a number imprinted on the handle and is labeled with an "L" for left or "R" for right. • Other forceps are designed according to the tooth morphology.

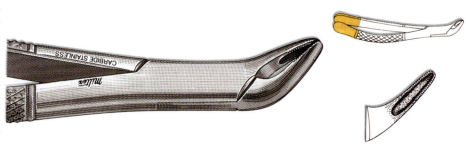

man incisors, cuspids,
and roots

#151 Mandibular Extraction Forceps

| **Use** | • Termed "universal forceps" |
| | • To remove mandibular incisors, cuspids, and roots |

Use
- Termed "universal forceps"
- To remove mandibular incisors, cuspids, and roots

Parts
- Handle
- Hinge
- Beak

Misc.
- Hinged instruments with various handles and beak styles
- Specific forceps are used on certain teeth or in certain areas of the mouth.
- Each instrument has a number imprinted on the handle and is labeled with an "L" for left or "R" for right.
- Other forceps are designed according to the tooth morphology.

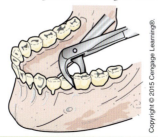

Copyright © 2015 Cengage Learning®.

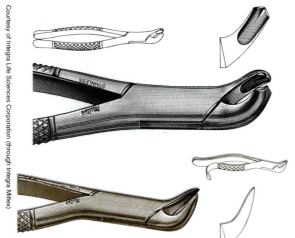

Man 1st 2nd
molars

#23 Universal Mandibular Extraction Forceps and #17 Universal Mandibular Extraction Forceps

Use	To remove first and second molars
Parts	• Handle • Hinge • Beak
Misc.	• Termed the "cow horn" forceps due to the bend of the beaks, with the point at the end of each beak. • Beaks have a formed point in the middle to go into the bifurcation (where the roots divide). • Available in right and left if the handle is curved (called the finger ring on the handle) • Hinged instruments with various handles and beak styles • Specific forceps are used on certain teeth or in certain areas of the mouth. • Each instrument has a number imprinted on the handle and is labeled with an "L" for left or "R" for right. • Other forceps are designed according to the tooth morphology.

Use

Parts

Misc.

To remove first and second molars

- Handle
- Hinge
- Beak

- Termed the "cow horn" forceps due to the bend of the beaks, with the point at the end of each beak.
- Beaks have a formed point in the middle to go into the bifurcation (where the roots divide).
- Available in right and left if the handle is curved (called the finger ring on the handle)
- Hinged instruments with various handles and beak styles
- Specific forceps are used on certain teeth or in certain areas of the mouth.
- Each instrument has a number imprinted on the handle and is labeled with an "L" for left or "R" for right.
- Other forceps are designed according to the tooth morphology.

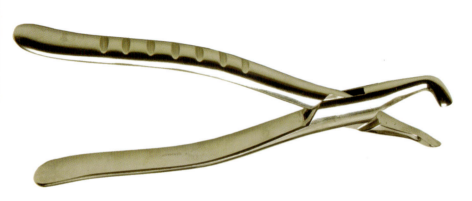

Man 3rd molars

#222 Mandibular Extraction Forceps

| **Use** | • Termed "universal" |
| | • Used to remove third molars |

Parts	• Handle
	• Hinge
	• Beak

Misc.	• Hinged instruments with various handles and beak styles
	• Specific forceps are used on certain teeth or in certain areas of the mouth.
	• Each instrument has a number imprinted on the handle and is labeled with an "L" for left or "R" for right.
	• Other forceps are designed according to the tooth morphology.

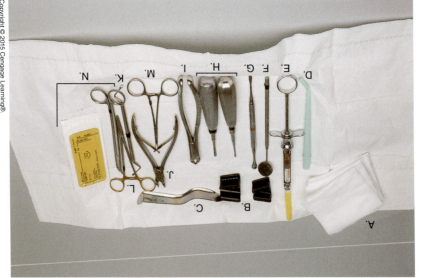

Tray Setup for Simple Extraction

A. Gauze sponges
B. Mouth props
C. Retractor for the tongue and the cheek
D. Surgical high-volume evacuator (HVE) tip
E. Local anesthetic
F. Mouth mirror
G. Periosteal elevator
H. Straight elevators
I. Extraction forceps
J. Rongeurs
K. Surgical curette
L. Needle Holder
M. Hemostat
N. Surgical Scissors/Suture setup

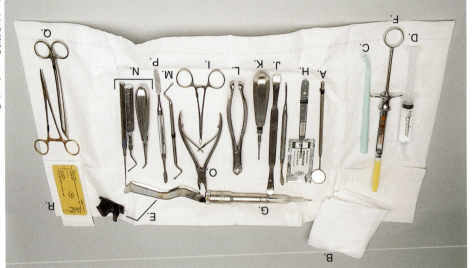

Tray Setup for Multiple Extractions and Alveoplasty

Parts

A. Mouth mirror
B. Gauze sponges
C. Surgical HVE tip
D. Luer Lock syringe and sterile saline solution
E. Retractor for the tongue and cheeks
F. Local anesthetic setup
G. Low-speed handpiece and surgical burs
H. Scalpel and blades
I. Hemostat and tissue retractors
J. Periosteal elevator
K. Straight elevator
L. Extraction forceps
M. Surgical curette
N. Elevators and Root Tip Pick
O. Rongeurs
P. Bone file
Q. Surgical Scissors and needle holder
R. Suture setup

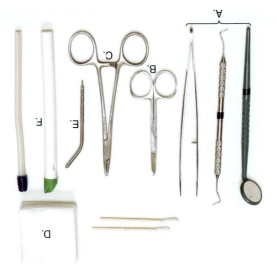

Tray Setup for Suture Removal

A. Basic setup, mouth mirror, explorer, cotton pliers
B. Suture scissors
C. Hemostat
D. Gauze sponges
E. Air-water syringe tip
F. HVE tip and/or saliva ejector

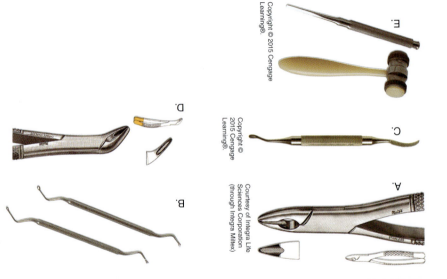

Test Your Knowledge

E.

Copyright © 2015 Cengage Learning®.

C.

Copyright © 2015 Cengage Learning®.

D.

Courtesy of Integra Life Sciences Corporation (through Integra Miltex)

B.

Copyright © 2015 Cengage Learning®.

A.

Courtesy of Integra Life Sciences Corporation (through Integra Miltex)

_____ 1. Identify the surgical curette.

_____ 2. Identify the surgical bone file.

_____ 3. Identify the mallet and the chisel.

_____ 4. Identify the forceps that are used to remove the lower molars.

_____ 5. Identify the forceps that are used to remove the maxillary incisors and cuspids.

Orthodontic Instruments

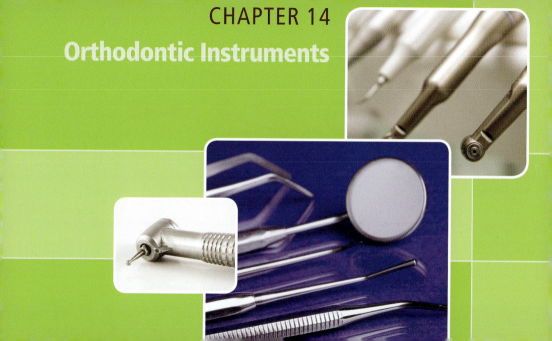

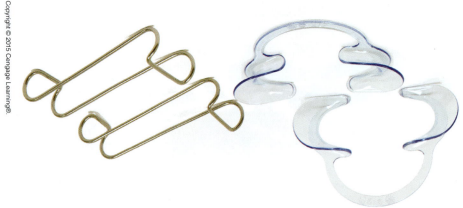

Orthodontic Lip and Cheek Retractors

Use	• To hold the lips and cheeks out of the way during orthodontic treatment
	• To retract the lips and cheeks out of the way during a photo shoot
Parts	Two U-shaped guards, connected or separate, that are placed at the corners of the patient's mouth to retract the tissue out of the way of the operator
Misc.	• Available in a variety of styles and sizes
	• Made from plastic or metal
	• Reusable (autoclavable) or disposable
	• Camera systems used in oral photography sometimes come with lip and cheek retractors.
	• Keeps the entire field in view and dry
	• Many retractors come with tabs or handles that the dental assistant or patient uses to hold back the lips and cheeks.
	• Some come with areas for the saliva ejector placement.

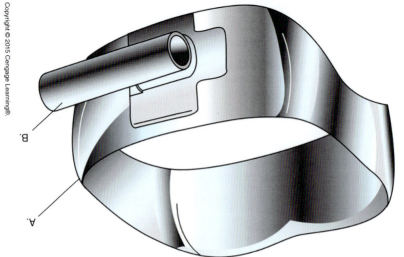

B.

A.

Orthodontic Bands

Use	• To cement around a tooth to hold and control tooth movement
	• Tubes, brackets, and attachments are fused and applied to the band to facilitate tooth movement.
	• Used for holding arch wires
	• For placement of the orthodontic headgear while patient is wearing it

Parts

A. Stainless steel band to be placed on posterior teeth
B. Bracket and buccal tube placed on the band

Misc.

- Come in a variety of sizes and are cemented in place
- Used on the posterior teeth
- Disposable
- Anatomically designed to fit the tooth
- Available in right and left anatomy and accurate gingival contouring

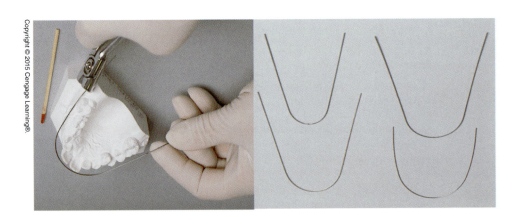

Orthodontic Arch Wire

Use	To apply force to either move the teeth or hold the desired positions
Parts	Nickel titanium or stainless steel arch wires that fit the natural arch form
Misc.	

- Secured to the brackets by ligature ties or elastics
- Supplied in different shapes: round, rectangular, etc.
- Supplied in different diameters and compositions, which alter the effect of the treatment
- Dispose of in sharps containers
- Placed in the buccal tubes and brackets that have been secured to the tooth
- Nickel titanium memory wire is designed to hold its shape.

Orthodontic Brackets and Bracket Trays

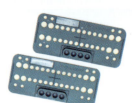

C.

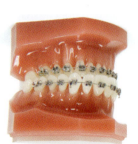

B.

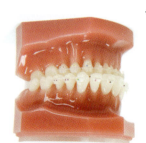

A.

Use	• To hold the arch wire in place
	• To transmit the force of the arch wire to move the teeth
	• Trays hold brackets and/or bands in order prior to their placement on the teeth.
Parts	• Anatomical brackets made to fit on the middle third of the teeth; each bracket has a slot to hold the arch wire.
	A. Clear brackets
	B. Metal brackets
	C. Compartmental trays to hold each bracket in anatomical order to prevent brackets from spilling
Misc.	• Brackets are either welded to the bands or bonded directly to the teeth.
	• Posterior brackets are made of stainless steel.
	• Anterior brackets are made of stainless steel, ceramic, or acrylic materials.
	• Some trays have adhesive backing to prevent spilling.

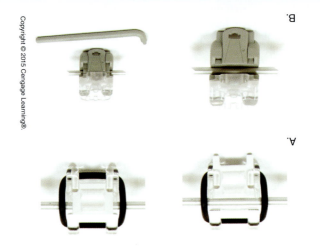

B.

A.

Self-Ligating Bracket System and Placement Instrument (Damon)

Use	To hold and secure the arch wire to the brackets without the use of ligature wire or elastics
Parts	**A.** Clear self-ligating Damon bracket with placement instrument
	B. Metal self-ligating Damon bracket
Misc.	• The bracket has a slot that opens for placement and removal of the arch wire.
	• The self-ligating bracket holds the arch wire tighter to control movement, therefore reducing treatment time.
	• Several styles of self-ligating brackets are available on the market.

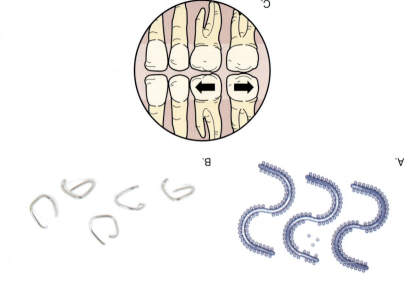

A.

B.

C.

Separators

Use	To separate the teeth to allow for placement of the orthodontic bands
Parts	**A.** Elastic separators that are placed in the contact area to force the teeth apart to accommodate the orthodontic band
	B. Metal C-shaped springs that are placed in the interproximal area to gently force the teeth apart for space for the orthodontic band
	C. Drawing showing how the teeth are spread after placement of elastic separators
Misc.	• A few days prior to band placement, the patient has the separators placed.
	• Many different elastic separators are available.
	• Many different-shaped metal separators are available.
	• Brass wire is also used for teeth separation.

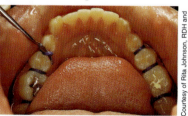

Courtesy of Rita Johnson, RDH and
Dr. Vincent DeAngelis

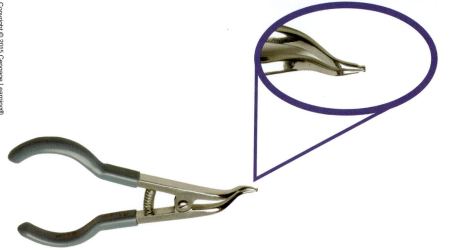

**Force Module Separating Pliers
(Elastic Separating Pliers)**

Use	To securely hold the elastic separators while placing them in the contact area between the teeth
Parts	• Hinged instrument with spring action • Small projections on each side to hold and grip the elastic separators • Single ended
Misc.	• Sterilized

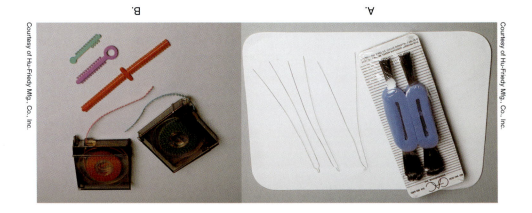

A.

B.

Courtesy of Hu-Friedy Mfg., Co., Inc.

Courtesy of Hu-Friedy Mfg., Co., Inc.

Orthodontic Ligature Wire/Elastic Modules

	To hold the arch wire to the brackets
Use	
Parts	**A.** Ligature wire is a very thin, flexible wire that comes in precut lengths or on spools.
	B. Elastic modules come in many colors to motivate patients to wear them, and come on sticks, canes, and chains.
Misc.	• Placed with the Coons ligature-tying pliers
	• The elastic modules may be placed with an explorer or scaler.
	• Sterilized

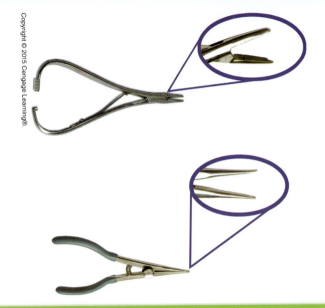

Coons Ligature-Tying Pliers and Mathieu Needle Holders

Use
- To manipulate and tie the ligature wire
- To place elastic ligatures
- To hold and place ligatures and separators

Parts
- A spring-loaded hinged instrument with two beaks at the working end; they are serrated for a tight grip.
- Each beak end is notched to hold the ligature wire.
- At the non-working end or handle is a locking device.

Misc.
- Available in a variety of styles
- Sterilized
- Also called an orthodontic hemostat
- One action will lock and release these pliers.

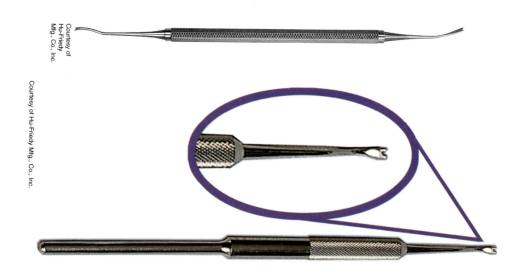

Ligature Director

Use	To tuck twisted ligature wire ends into the interproximal spaces
Parts	A single- or double-ended instrument with the working end notched for placement of the ligature.
Misc.	• Available in different types of working ends, with some resembling a plugger or scaler • The working ends of the instrument are notched to secure and manipulate the ligature wire around the brackets. • Sterilized

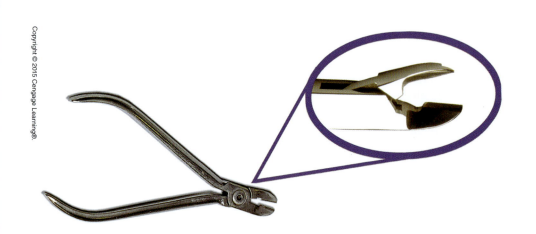

Pin and Ligature Cutter or Light Cutting Pliers

Use	To cut thin ligature wire during placement and removal of orthodontic arch wire
Parts	• A hinged instrument with cutting blade on working end • Photo shows the back of the entire instrument with a close-up of the working-end top side.
Misc.	• Available in various sizes and shapes • Available in straight, angled, or tapered working ends

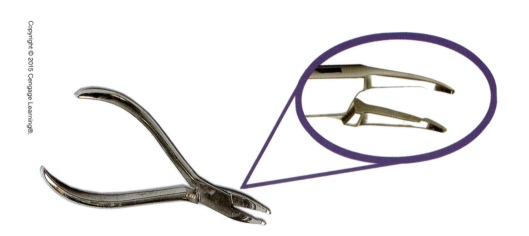

How (Howe) Pliers/Utility Pliers

- To manipulate, place, and remove the arch wire
- To check for loose appliances

Parts

- A hinged plier with serrated beaks
- Photo shows the back of the entire instrument with a close-up of the working-end top side

Misc.

- Curved or straight beaks
- The working ends are flat and serrated for tighter grip.

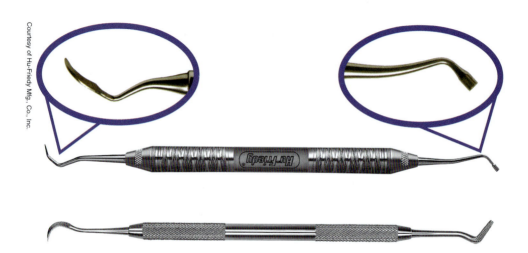

Courtesy of Hu-Friedy Mfg. Co., Inc.

Band Seater/Plugger with Scaler

| **Use** | • To place or seat posterior orthodontic bands |
| | • To remove excess cement |

Parts A straight double-ended instrument with an angled scaler on one end and an angled condenser on the other end

Misc.
- Double ended
- Various shapes of condensers are available.
- Various types of scalers are available.
- Serrated plugger on one end and a sharp scaler on the other end

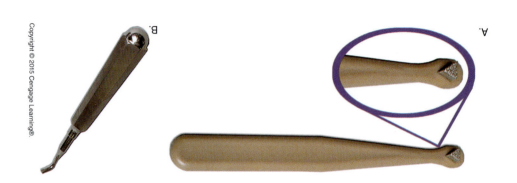

Bite Stick/Band Seater and Band Pusher

A.

B.

| **Use** | • To seat the orthodontic bands during the try-in and cementation appointments |
| | • To push the orthodontic band into place during the try-in and cementation appointments |

Parts

A. The bite stick is a straight plastic broad instrument with a triangular metal serrated insert on the working end. On the opposite side of the insert is a wide flat surface.

B. The band pusher is a large-handled metal instrument with a tapered angled working end. The working end has a flat serrated tip.

Misc.

• Uses force of occlusion to seat the band
• Also called a band biter
• Single ended
• Flat stick with small metal triangle on the working end that sits on the orthodontic band; the patient then bites down on the flat opposite side.
• The band pusher has large handle for good grip to apply pressure on the orthodontic band.

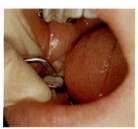

Courtesy of Rita Johnson, RDH and Dr. Vincent DeAngelis

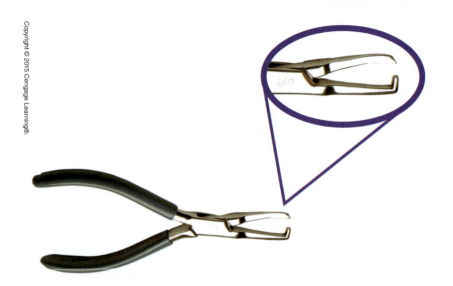

Posterior Band-Removing Pliers

Use	To remove posterior orthodontic bands from the teeth
Parts	A hinged plier with different-shaped working ends: One beak has a round plastic cover to place on the occlusal surface of the teeth; the other beak has a small flat surface that is placed under the band near the gingival tissue or under the bracket on the band.
Misc.	• Pressure is applied and the band is gently removed from the tooth. • Some band-removing pliers have replaceable plastic tips.

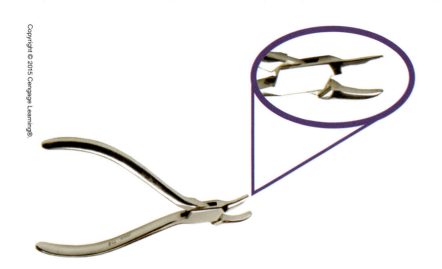

Band-Contouring Pliers

Use	To crimp and re-form crowns and orthodontic bands to adapt more tightly to the tooth
Parts	A hinged plier with beaks that curve and contour at the same plane
Misc.	• One beak is rounded and blunt ended.
	• Sometimes called crown- and band-crimping pliers
	• The other beak has a notch where the beaks fit together.
	• The band fits between the beaks to be shaped and contoured.

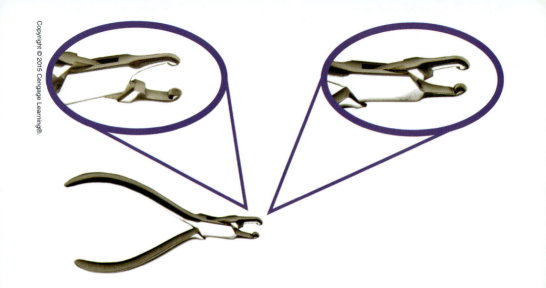

Contouring Ball Pliers

| **Use** | • To contour orthodontic bands |
| | • To contour stainless steel/aluminum crowns |

Parts   A hinged instrument with beaks; one is a ball and the other is a matching socket.

Misc.   • Matched ball and socket tips for contouring the bands
             • Large and small tips are available.

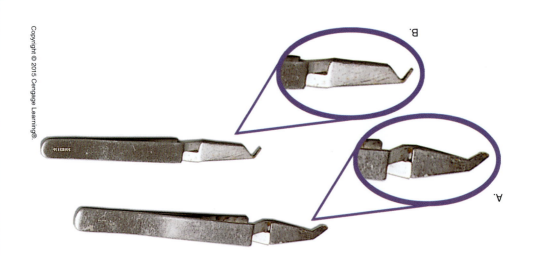

B.

A.

Bracket Forceps

Use
- To hold and pass the brackets for placement and positioning
- To place the brackets on the tooth for bonding

Parts
The instrument has handles that you pinch together to allow the tips to secure and release the brackets.

A. Posterior bracket forceps
B. Anterior bracket forceps

Misc.
- Range of sizes and shapes

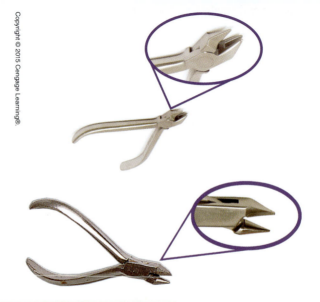

Bird-Beak Pliers and Three-Prong Pliers

<table>
<tr><td>**Use**</td><td>

- To contour and bend wire, clasps, and loops
- To form springs in orthodontic wire
- To adjust wire on retainers and other appliances with wire

</td></tr>
<tr><td>**Parts**</td><td>

A hinged instrument that has two short working ends: One of the working ends is triangular in shape; the other working end is rounded in shape (bird beak). One side has only one beak and the other side has two beaks (three-prong).

</td></tr>
<tr><td>**Misc.**</td><td>

- The working ends are short beaks that meet precisely.
- Also referred to as the three-jaw plier (three-prong)
- Very strong pliers (three-prong)

</td></tr>
</table>

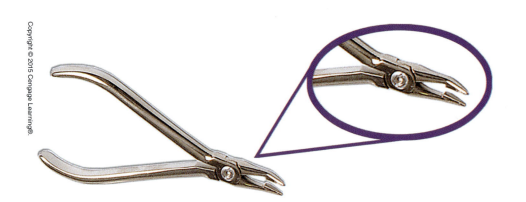

Weingart Utility Pliers

Use	• To place and remove arch wire
	• Used for numerous other orthodontic functions
Parts	A hinged instrument with elongated serrated clasping tips
Misc.	• Is slim enough to fit between the bracket and the arch wire
	• Very functional in manipulating orthodontic arch wire
	• The working ends are serrated and tapered.

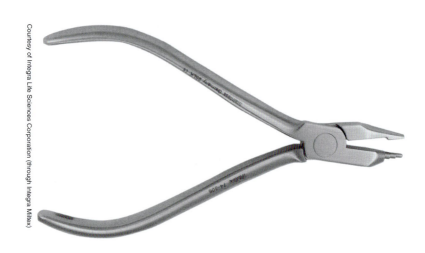

Tweed-Loop Pliers

Use	• To form loops and springs in the arch wire
	• To bend wires in removable appliances
Parts	A hinged instrument with two beaks: One beak has grooves in a graduated cone that assist in the bending of the wire and in forming the loops; the other beak is a flat serrated tip.
Misc.	• Variety of styles

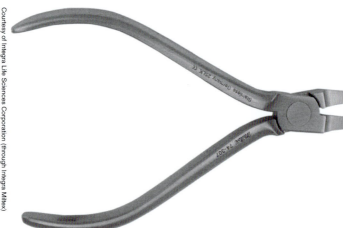

Arch-Bending Pliers

Use	• To bend arch wires
	• Designed for placing first-, second-, and, third-order bends
Parts	A hinged instrument with two tapered ends that are flat
Misc.	• One action will lock and release these pliers.
	• Available in a variety of styles

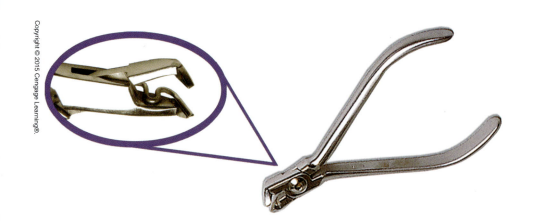

Distal End-Cutting Pliers

Use	• To cut the distal ends of the arch wire after the wire has been placed and secured in the brackets and the buccal tubes
	• Designed to grasp the cut end of the wire
Parts	A hinged instrument that has two beaks, one for cutting and the other for grasping the cut wire
Misc.	• A plastic bracket attaches to the pliers to catch the excess wire so it will not go down the patient's throat.
	• The pliers is designed to fit at the distal of the most posterior tooth at a right angle.
	• The pliers has a sharp edge to cut the excess arch wire.

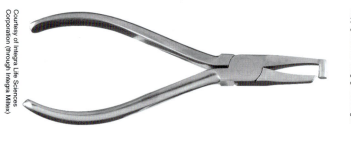

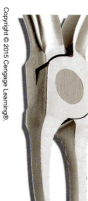

Bracket Removers and Adhesive-Removing Pliers

Use	• To remove brackets from the teeth
	• To remove excess adhesive from the tooth after the brackets have been removed
Parts	• Bracket removers are hinged instruments with two beaks that have sharp right-angle edges.
	• Adhesive-removing pliers are hinged instruments; one end has a plastic cap on it and the other working end is a flat surface.
Misc.	• The bracket remover has beaks that come together in a flat pointed edge to fit under the bracket and pry it loose.
	• Bracket removers are available in anterior, where the tips are straight, and posterior, where the tips are at a right angle.
	• Adhesive-removing pliers have two ends: One end of the pliers has a plastic pad that can be changed; the other end of the pliers has a short, straight beak to scrape off the adhesive.

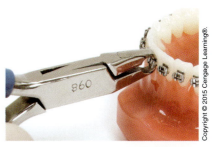

Copyright © 2015 Cengage Learning®.

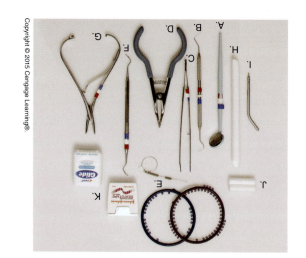

Tray Setup for Placement and Removal of Elastic Separators

Parts

A. Mouth mirror
B. Explorer
C. Cotton pliers
D. Separating pliers
E. Separators (elastic or metal separating materials)
F. Orthodontic scaler
G. Mathieu pliers
H. High-volume evacuator (HVE) tip
I. Air-water syringe tip
J. Cotton rolls
K. Dental floss or tape

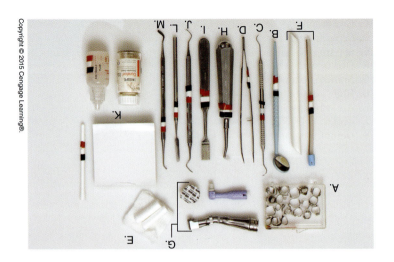

Tray Setup for Cementation of Orthodontic Bands

Parts

A. Selection of bands
B. Mouth mirror
C. Explorer
D. Cotton pliers
E. Cotton rolls and 2 × 2 gauze
F. Saliva ejector and HVE
G. Slow-speed handpiece with rubber cup and prophy paste
H. Band pusher
I. Bite stick/band seater
J. Scaler
K. Cement of choice, dispenser for powder, and paper pad
L. Cement spatula
M. Plastic filling instrument

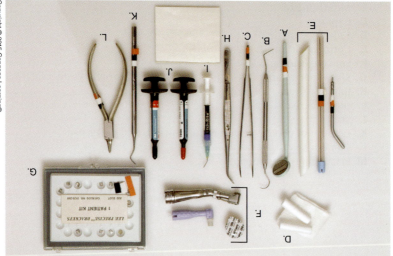

Tray Setup for Direct Bonding of Brackets

A. Mouth mirror
B. Explorer
C. Cotton pliers
D. Cotton rolls and 2 × 2 gauze
E. Air-water syringe tip, saliva ejector, and HVE
F. Contra-angle attachment or disposable prophy cup and prophy paste
G. Bracket kit
H. Locking cotton pliers
I. Etchant
J. Bonding agent
K. Scaler
L. Bird-beak pliers

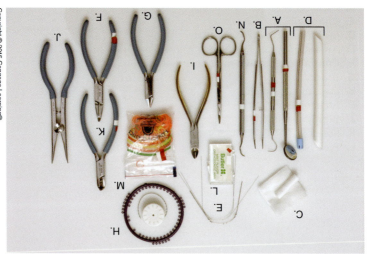

Tray Setup for Placement of Arch Wire and Ligature Ties

Parts

A. Mouth mirror, explorer
B. Cotton pliers
C. Cotton rolls and 2×2 gauze
D. HVE and saliva ejector
E. Selected arch wire
F. Weingart pliers
G. Bird-beak pliers
H. Elastics or ligature wire
I. Ligature-wire-cutting pliers
J. Ligature-tying pliers
K. Distal end-cutting pliers
L. Orthodontic wax
M. Rubber bands
N. Orthodontic scaler
O. Scissors

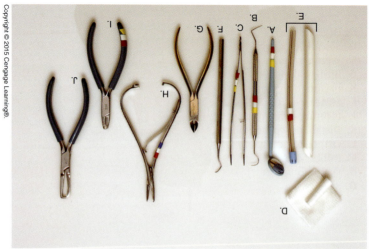

Tray Setup for Appliance Removal Appointment

Parts

- **A.** Mouth mirror
- **B.** Explorer
- **C.** Cotton pliers
- **D.** Cotton rolls and 2×2 gauze
- **E.** HVE and saliva ejector
- **F.** Orthodontic scaler
- **G.** Ligature-wire-cutting pliers
- **H.** Mathieu pliers
- **I.** Bracket remover and adhesive-removing pliers
- **J.** Posterior band remover

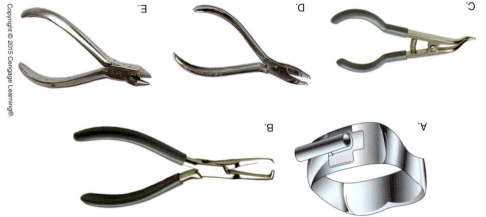

E.

D.

C.

B.

A.

Test Your Knowledge

_____ 1. Which pliers is used to stretch the elastics to place them in the contact area of the tooth?

_____ 2. Which instrument is used to place, manipulate, and remove ligature wire?

_____ 3. Brackets and buccal tubes are placed on these for orthodontic treatment.

_____ 4. Which instrument is used to contour wire and form springs in orthodontic wire?

_____ 5. Which instrument is used to remove the posterior orthodontic bands from the teeth?

Pedodontic Instruments

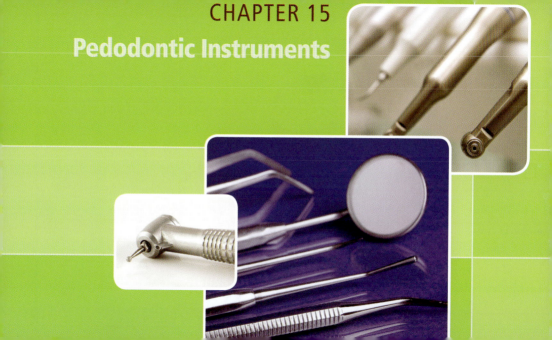

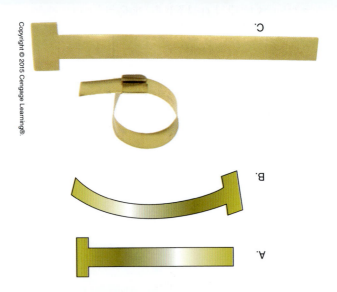

T-Band Matrix

A.

B.

C.

Use	Used on primary teeth to establish the normal contour of the prepared tooth while the tooth is being filled with the restorative material

Parts	• Brass strips that are "crossed" at one end
	   A. Straight
	   B. Curved
	   C. Straight T-Band shown made into a ring, ready to apply.

Misc.	• Available in various designs and sizes • Do not require retainers • Are adjustable • Can be secured on the tooth by bending the "T" extensions at a right angle to the strip and by sliding the strip through it to make a ring that can be pulled tighter on the tooth

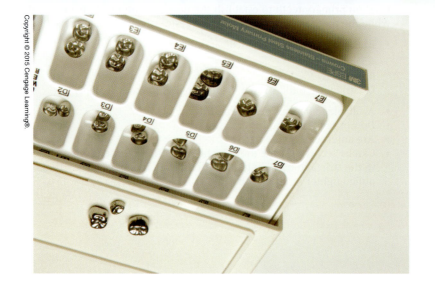

Stainless Steel Crown Kit

Use	• To replace tooth structure when there have been extensive carious lesions
	• To replace tooth structure when there are hypoplastic or hypocalcified teeth
	• To replace tooth structure following a pulpotomy or pulpectomy
	• To be used as an abutment tooth for a space-maintainer
	• To be used as a temporary restoration for a fractured tooth
Parts	Anatomical stainless steel crowns in various sizes
Misc.	• Available in a variety of sizes and can be purchased individually or in a kit

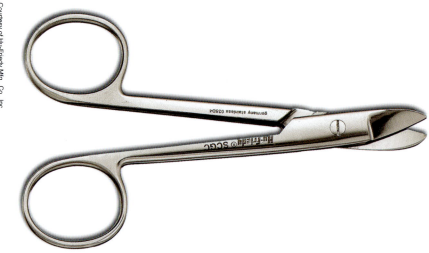

Crown and Collar Scissors

Use
- To trim aluminum temporary crowns on the gingival area
- To trim stainless steel crowns on the gingival area
- To cut gingival retraction cord
- To trim custom provisional restorations
- To trim matrix bands

Parts
- Hinged scissors with enclosed circle handles that can be manipulated with one hand
- Cutting beaks available in straight or curved tips

Misc.
- Available in narrow or wide cutting edges
- Available in a variety of sizes

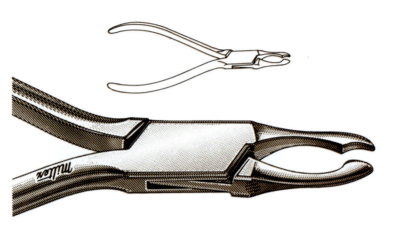

Courtesy of Integra Life Sciences Corporation (through Integra Miltex)

miltex

Contouring and Crimping Pliers

Use	To crimp and contour the marginal edge of the aluminum or stainless steel crown
Parts	• Hinged instrument • Beaks: One has a convex surface and the other one has a concave surface that fits over the convex one.
Misc.	• Available in a range of sizes and shapes • The Johnson is a commonly used type of contouring pliers.

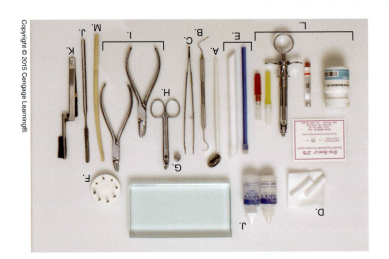

Tray Setup for Pediatric Stainless Steel Crown Placement

A. Mouth mirror
B. Expro
C. Cotton pliers
D. Cotton rolls and gauze
E. High-volume evacuator (HVE) and saliva ejector
F. High-speed handpiece (not shown) and selected burs
G. Stainless steel crown
H. Crown and collar scissors
I. Contouring and crimping pliers
J. Mixing spatula, paper pad, permanent cement
K. Articulating forceps and paper
L. Topical anesthetic, syringe, carpules, needles, Stick Shield
M. Orangewood stick

Not Shown

- Low-speed handpiece with green stone and rubber abrasive wheel
- Spoon excavator
- Dental floss

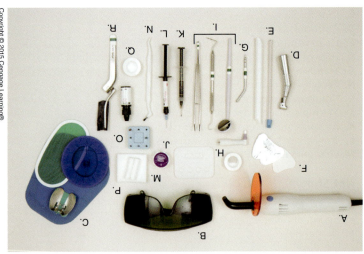

Tray Setup for Dental Sealant

A. Curing light
B. Protective glasses
C. Dental dam setup
D. Low-speed handpiece
E. Saliva ejector and HVE tip
F. Dry angle
G. Air-water syringe tip
H. Prophy angle with prophy paste without fluoride
I. Basic setup: mirror, explorer, and cotton pliers
J. Dispensing tray
K. Etchant
L. Sealant
M. Dental floss
N. Applicator brush
O. Bur block with assorted burs and/or stones
P. Cotton rolls and gauze
Q. Dappen dish and bonding agent
R. Articulating forceps with paper

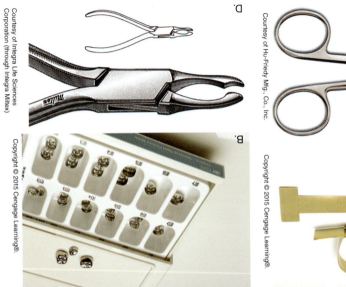

D.

C.

B.

A.

_____ 1. Which instrument is used to crimp and contour the marginal edge of the aluminum or stainless steel crown?

_____ 2. This item comes in brass in either straight or curved.

_____ 3. This kit has crowns to replace tooth structure.

_____ 4. This kit has crowns to be used as a temporary restoration for a fractured tooth.

_____ 5. Identify the crown and collar scissors.

Periodontic Instruments

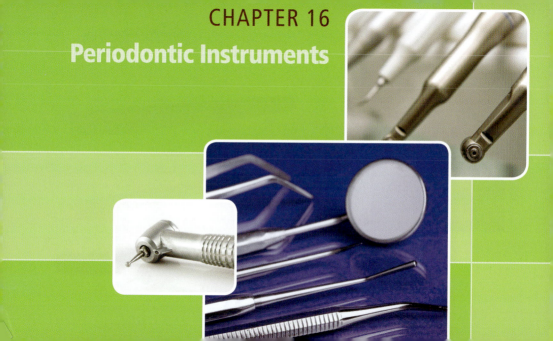

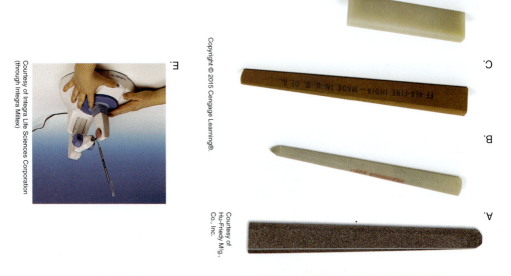

D.

C.

B.

A.

E.

FF 464-FINE INDIA–MADE IN U.S. OF A.

| **Use** | • To sharpen the cutting edges of periodontal instruments |
| | • To improve the effectiveness of the instruments |

Parts
- Manual sharpening stones come in several sizes and shapes.
- They are made of various materials, including: Arkansas stone, India oilstone, silicon carbide, and ceramic stones.
- The mechanical method for sharpening periodontal instruments is shown here.

A. Silicon carbide sharpening stone in cone shape
B. Ceramic sharpening stone in triangle shape
C. India sharpening stone
D. Arkansas sharpening stone
E. Mechanical sharpening device

Misc.
- Mechanical devices provide a consistent and precise sharpening method.
- Sometimes a lubricant is used when sharpening the instruments.
- Sharpening periodontal instruments requires training and practice.

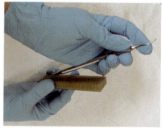

Copyright © 2015 Cengage Learning®.

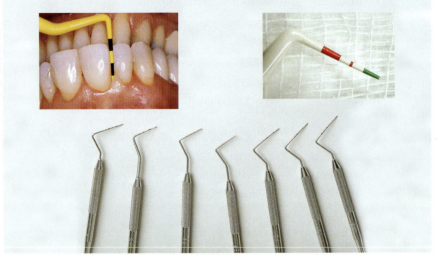

Periodontal Probes

Use	• To measure the depth of periodontal pockets in millimeters
	• To measure areas of recession, bleeding, or exudate

Parts   Calibrated instrument with a blunted working end

Misc.
- Probe may be flat, oval, or round in cross section but is thin enough to fit in the gingival sulcus.
- Many styles and variations in the millimeter markings
- The calibrations may be indentations or color coded for easy reading.
- May be double ended with probe on one end and an explorer on the other end
- Computerized probe systems detect and store information on pocket depth, recession, furcation involvement, and mobility.

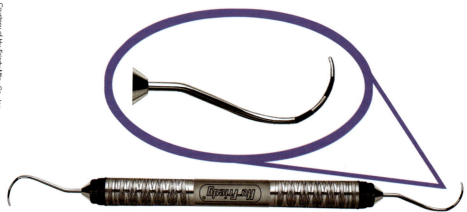

Furcation Probe

Use	To measure the pocket depth in furcation areas on multi-rooted teeth
Parts	An instrument with a rounded calibrated working end
Misc.	• Blunted or rounded ends • Can be single or double ended • Curved working ends with millimeter markings/calibrations • Markings may be indented or color coded.

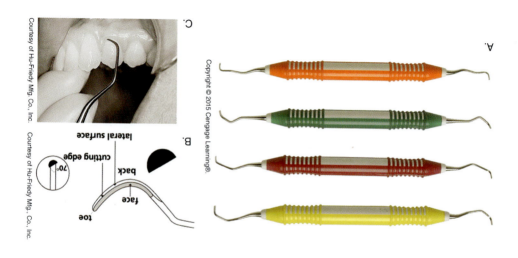

A.

Copyright © 2015 Cengage Learning®.

B.

toe
face
back
lateral surface
cutting edge
70°

Courtesy of Hu-Friedy Mfg. Co., Inc.

C.

Courtesy of Hu-Friedy Mfg. Co., Inc.

Periodontal Curettes

Use	• To remove subgingival calculus
	• To smooth the root surface in root planing
	• To remove the soft tissue lining or the periodontal pocket
	• Designed to adapt to the curves of the root surface

Parts
- A double-ended instrument where the working ends have a cutting edge on one or both sides of the blade
- The end of the instrument is rounded, not pointed like a scaler.

A. Variety of anterior and posterior curettes
B. Drawing of the working end of a curette
C. Curette being used in oral cavity

Misc.
- Many types of curettes exist, including the universal and Gracey, which are designed and angled to be used in specific areas of the mouth, such as the anterior and posterior.
- Handles may be color coded and ergonomically designed.
- Mainly double ended
- Available in a range of sizes, usually 1/2, 3/4, and so on, with the size label following the manufacturer's name
- Often named for designer, for example, Gracey, McCalls, or Langer

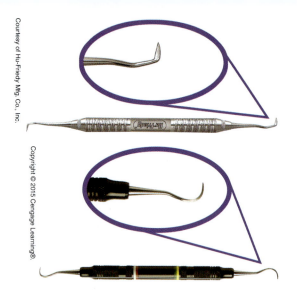

Periodontal Scaler: Sickle and Jacquette

Use

To remove supragingival calculus

Parts

- An instrument with working ends that have two cutting edges along the margins of the curved blade; the end of the instrument is a sharp point.
- There are three angles in the shank of the instrument (Jacquette).

Misc.

- The periodontal scaler is also known as the shepherd's hook.
- Single and doubled ended
- The sickle scaler looks like the agricultural tool called a sickle.
- Variety of sizes and angles
- The Jacquette is able to get closer to the root to remove the calculus.

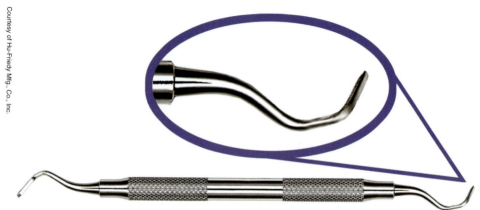

Courtesy of Hu-Friedy Mfg. Co., Inc.

Periodontal Chisel Scaler

Use	To remove supragingival and subgingival deposits from the root of the tooth
Parts	• The working end is a blade that is slightly curved and the cutting edge is beveled. • There are two angles in the shank.
Misc.	• Available in a variety of sizes and shapes • Single and double ended • Some have a broader blade at the working end.

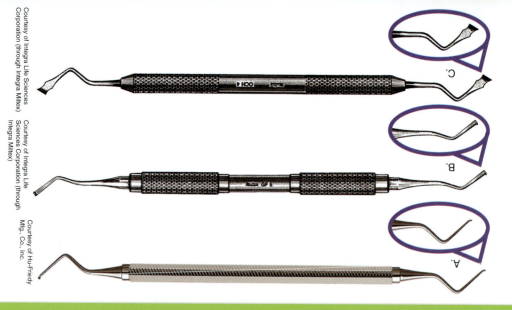

Periodontal Hoe Scalers

A.

Courtesy of Hu-Friedy Mfg. Co., Inc.

B.

Courtesy of Integra Life Sciences Corporation (through Integra Miltex)

C.

Courtesy of Integra Life Sciences Corporation (through Integra Miltex)

| **Use** | • To remove supragingival and subgingival calculus from around the tooth |
| | • To plane and smooth the root surface |

| **Parts** | An instrument that resembles the agricultural hoe tool and has a straight cutting edge |

A. Mesial/distal hoe
B. Buccal/lingual hoe
C. Back-action hoe

Misc.	• Used in a pulling motion
	• Double- or single-ended instrument
	• Variety of sizes and designs

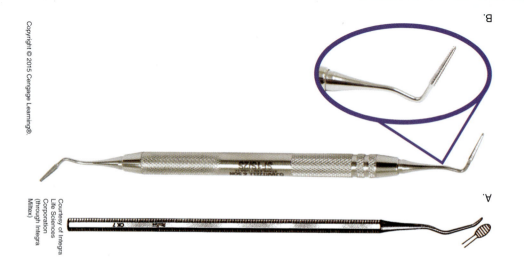

B.

A.

Courtesy of Integra
Life Sciences
Corporation
(through Integra
Miltex)

Periodontal Files

| **Use** | • To accomplish root planing |
| | • To remove supragingival and subgingival calculus from the interproximal surface |

Parts An instrument that has a long neck with cutting groves on the working end

A. Double-ended periodontal file
B. Double-ended interproximal periodontal file

Misc.	• Variety of blade shapes and shank angulations
	• Pushing and pulling motion interproximally
	• Some are designed with a long grooved working end to be used interproximately.
	• Various sizes and shapes

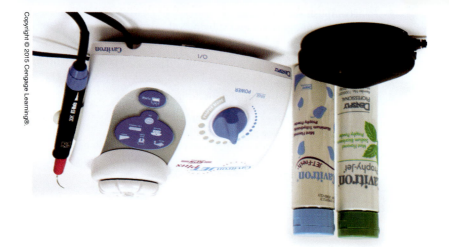

Ultrasonic Scaler and Air Polishing Unit (Cavitron®)

Use	• To remove hard deposits, stains, and debris during scaling, curettage, and root planing procedures
	• To polish surfaces more thoroughly than by conventional means
	• To clean tooth surfaces prior to bonding procedures and placing of sealants

Use

- To remove hard deposits, stains, and debris during scaling, curettage, and root planing procedures
- To polish surfaces more thoroughly than by conventional means
- To clean tooth surfaces prior to bonding procedures and placing of sealants

Parts

A combined ultrasonic scaler and air polishing unit that has a handpiece for use with scaling tips as well as a foot control that controls the speed of the unit. It has an air polishing insert (sodium bicarbonate, air, and water).

Misc.

- Comes with a variety of tips
- The air polisher delivers a mixture of sodium bicarbonate, air, and water to polish the teeth.
- Various sizes and types of ultrasonic and air polishing units are available; they can be purchased as independent units.
- Foot controls can be wireless.
- The ultrasonic unit generates high-power vibrations to a handpiece with a variety of tips.
- Ultrasonic units cause heat, so the units have cooling systems that circulate water through the handpieces and out the openings near the tips.

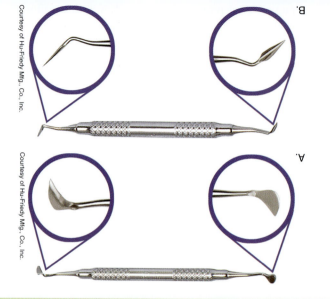

B.

A.

Periodontal Knives and Interdental Knives

| **Use** | • Periodontal knives remove and contour gingival tissue during periodontal surgery. |
| | • Interdental knives interproximally remove soft tissue. |

| **Parts** | **A.** The periodontal knife is an instrument with a round-bladed working end with cutting edges. |
| | **B.** The interdental knife is a spear-shaped instrument with long, narrow blades. |

Misc.	• The most common periodontal knives are kidney-shaped and broad-bladed knives.
	• The entire periphery of the blade is sharp.
	• Single and doubled ended
	• Periodontal knives are also called gingivectomy knives.
	• Common designer names: Kirkland, Buck, Goldman-Fox (periodontal)
	• Common designer names: Orban, Goldman-Fox (interdental)

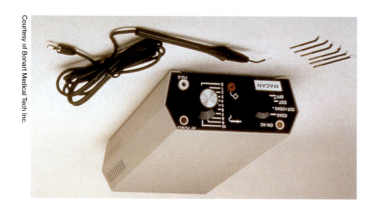

Courtesy of Bonart Medical Tech Inc.

Electrosurgery Unit

| **Use** | • To incise and contour gingival tissue |
| | • To coagulate the blood during surgical procedures |

Parts
- Control box
- Two terminal plates: One is placed behind the patient's back or shoulders and the other is a probe with various cutting tips that is used during surgery.
- Foot-operated on/off controls
- The electrosurgery unit uses timed electrical currents to incise the tissue.

Misc.
- A dental assistant must keep the high-volume evacuator (HVE) close during the use of the electrosurgery unit to remove debris and odor.
- Many tips are available.

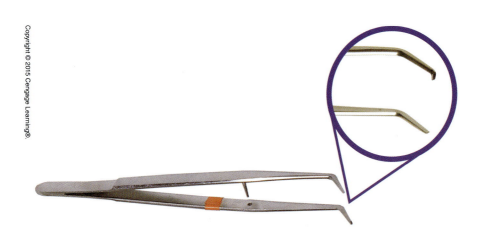

Pocket-Marking Pliers

| **Use** | To transfer the measurement of the pocket to the outside of the tissue to indicate the depth level of the pocket |

Use

To transfer the measurement of the pocket to the outside of the tissue to indicate the depth level of the pocket

Parts

Pliers that have one straight thin beak that is placed in the pocket; the other beak is bent at a right angle at the tip.

Misc.

- When the beaks are pinched together, the gingival tissue is perforated, which leaves small pinpoint markings.
- It resembles a cotton pliers, but the tips are different.

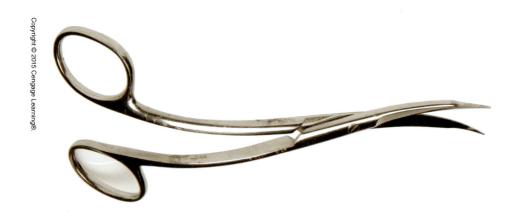

Periodontal Scissors

Use	• To remove tags of tissue and to trim margins of tissue
	• Also used in oral maxillofacial surgeries and endodontic procedures
Parts	Scissors with long, very thin and sharp blades
Misc.	• Many varieties of shapes and sizes

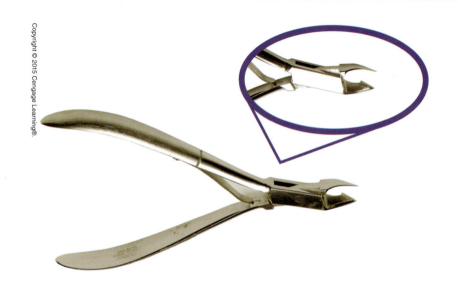

Periodontal Rongeurs

Use	To remove excess tissue and to shape the soft tissue
Parts	Hinged pliers with sharp cutting edge on one side of the blade of the working end
Misc.	• Smaller than bone rongeurs • Periodontal rongeurs are also known as nippers.

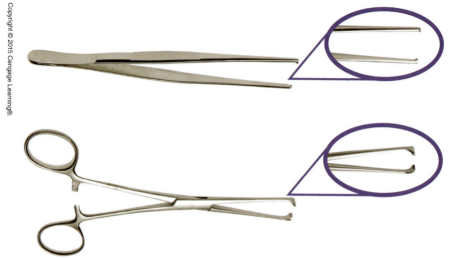

Periodontal Forceps

Use	• To retract soft tissue during surgical procedures
	• To hold soft tissue in place
Parts	An instrument with beaks that are often curved near the end at right angles to each other; the ends are sharp to securely hold the tissue.
	A. Hinged locking tissue forceps
	B. Cotton-plier-designed tissue forceps with tongue and groove ends
Misc.	• Many varieties of shapes and designs
	• They are shaped like cotton pliers or hemostats with locking handles.

B.

A.

Periotomes

Use	• To sever the periodontal ligament prior to extraction
	• To use to prepare for dental implants
Parts	An instrument with flexible fixed blades that are thin, sharp, and designed to cause minimal damage to the periodontal ligament
	A. Posterior periotomes
	B. Anterior periotomes
Misc.	• Single or double ended
	• Straight or angled blade
	• Various sizes and shapes
	• Made of stainless steel
	• Available with handle and interchangeable blades
	• Available in wide, narrow, angled, and contra-angled blades

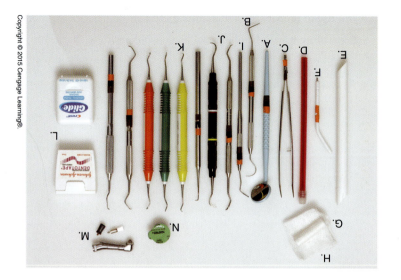

Tray Setup for Scaling, Curettage, and Polish Procedure

Parts

A. Mouth mirror
B. Explorer
C. Cotton pliers
D. Saliva ejector
E. High-volume evacuation (HVE) tip
F. Air-water syringe tip
G. Cotton rolls
H. Gauze sponges
I. Periodontal probe
J. Scalers: Jacquette and shepherd's hook
K. Curettes: universal and Gracey
L. Dental floss and tape
M. Prophy angle: rubber cups and brushes
N. Prophy paste

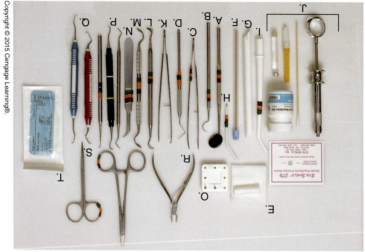

Tray Setup for Gingivectomy Procedure

A. Mouth mirror
B. Explorer
C. Cotton pliers
D. Periodontal probe
E. Cotton rolls and gauze sponges
F. Saliva ejector
G. HVE tip
H. Air-water syringe tip
I. Surgical aspirating tip
J. Anesthetic setup
K. Pocket marker
L. Periodontal knives
M. Interproximal knives
N. Scalpel and blade
O. Diamond burs
P. Scalers
Q. Curettes
R. Soft tissue rongeurs
S. Hemostat and surgical scissors
T. Suture needle and thread

Not shown: Periodontal dressing materials

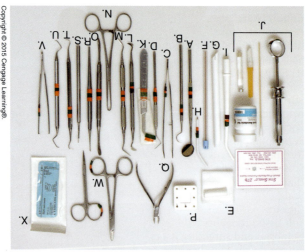

Tray Setup for Osseous Surgery

Parts

A. Mouth mirror
B. Explorer
C. Cotton pliers
D. Periodontal probe
E. Cotton rolls and gauze sponges
F. Saliva ejector
G. HVE tip
H. Air-water syringe tip
I. Surgical aspirating tip
J. Anesthetic setup
K. Scalpel and blade
L. Broad-bladed periodontal knife
M. Interproximal periodontal knife

N. Tissue retractor
O. Periosteal elevator
P. Diamond burs and stones
Q. Periodontal rongeurs
R. Chisels
S. Files
T. Scalers
U. Curettes
V. Tissue forceps
W. Scissors
X. Suture setup

Not shown: Periodontal dressing materials

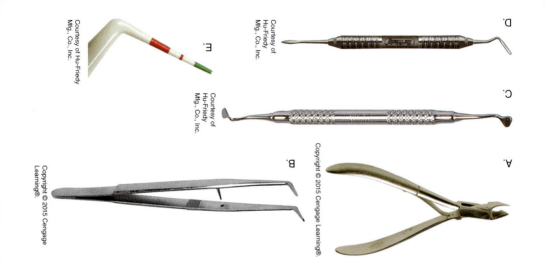

_____ 1. This calibrated instrument is used to measure periodontal pockets.

_____ 2. Which instrument is also called a gingivectomy knife and is used to remove and contour gingival tissue during periodontal surgery?

_____ 3. Which instrument is used to sever the periodontal ligament before an extraction?

_____ 4. Which instrument is used to remove and contour gingival tissue during periodontal surgery and is also called "nippers"?

_____ 5. Which instrument is used to transfer the measurement of the pocket to the outside of the tissue to indicate the depth level of the pocket before surgery?

Fixed Prosthodontic Instruments

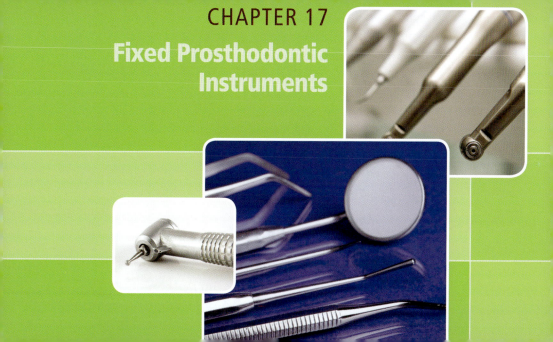

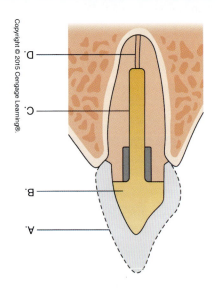

Core Post

A.

B.

C.

D.

Use	• To support and provide retention for the restoration
	• A post-retained core is used when the tooth is non-vital.
	• The root canal filling is removed and the post is fitted in the canal and cemented.
Parts	• Drill to make the desired preparation
	• Wrenches or keys for hand placement of the core post

A. Crown of the tooth
B. Core buildup
C. Core post
D. Apical seal of root canal

Misc.
- Available in different sizes
- Often purchased as a kit
- After being fitted in the root canal, it is cemented in place.
- Made from materials such as titanium, titanium alloy, and stainless steel

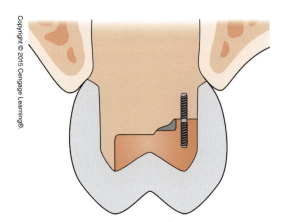

Retention Pins

| **Use** | • For addition or retention of the core buildup material |
| | • For support and retention of a restoration |

Parts	• Drills to be used in the low-speed handpiece to drill holes for the specific retention pins
	• Hand driver or mechanical placement device
	• Pins

| **Misc.** | • Often come in kits |

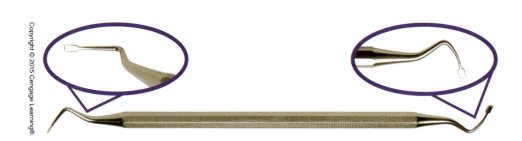

Retraction Cord Placement Instrument

Use

To place retraction cord around a prepared tooth so that the tissue is displaced and ready for an accurate and detailed impression

Parts

- Single- or double-ended instrument
- If double ended, the ends are angled differently and can have different working ends.

Misc.

- Working ends can have smooth or serrated edges.
- Available in a variety of sizes and shapes
- Other instruments can be utilized for placing retraction cord, such as explorers, spoon excavators, periodontal probes, and so forth.

Cement Mixing Spatula

To mix dental cements and materials

Single-ended flat spatula and handle

- The spatula is flexible or rigid and allows proper manipulation of materials.
- Made of stainless steel
- Sterilized
- The edge of the spatula can be used to gather the materials for use.
- Available in a range of sizes

Wooden Bite Stick

Use	To aid in seating the permanent crown during adaptation and cementation
Parts	Wooden bite stick, also known as an orangewood stick; 6 inches long and 3/16 in round diameter
Misc.	• Comes in a range of different sizes • Made of soft wood

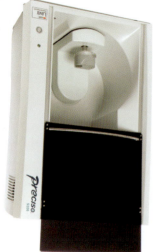

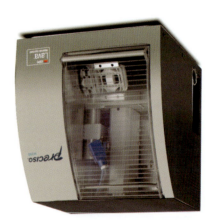

Computer-Aided Design (CAD)

Use	• Used to obtain a virtual impression of the teeth
	• Transmits the obtained information to the dental laboratory for its use (e.g., to construct crowns, etc.)

Parts A computer unit that captures images digitally with either a video camera or a laser camera. It saves the image so the operator can transmit it to the dental laboratory. It has a handheld scanner that is placed into the oral cavity to obtain the image.

• LAVA COS system

Misc.
• iTero and LAVA are types of CAD systems.
• Information is sent to manufacture the model, and then a model is sent to the laboratory.
• Some units require powder on the teeth to obtain the impression.

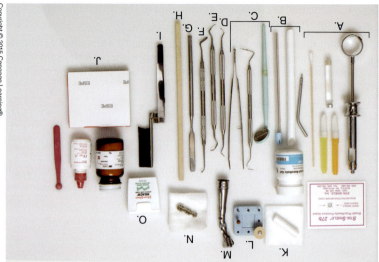

Tray Setup for the Crown Cementation Appointment

Use	This tray is set up when the patient comes into the office for the final crown or bridge to be cemented over the prepared tooth.
Parts	**A.** Anesthetic syringe, needles, carpule, cotton-tip applicator, topical anesthetic, and Stik-Shield
	B. Three-way syringe tip, high-volume evacuator (HVE) tip, saliva ejector
	C. Basic setup: mouth mirror, expro (explorer and periodontal probe combination), cotton pliers
	D. Spoon excavator
	E. Curette
	F. Plastic instrument
	G. Mixing spatula
	H. Wood bite stick
	I. Articulation paper and holder
	J. Final cementation materials
	K. Cotton roll and gauze
	L. Miscellaneous burs
	M. Latch-type contra-angle
	N. Bridge ready for cementation
	O. Dental floss

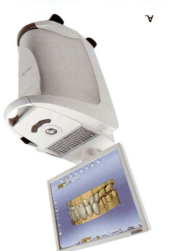

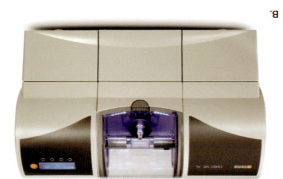

A.

B.

Computer-Aided Design (CAD) and Computer-Aided Manufacturing (CAM) Systems

Use	• Used to obtain a virtual impression of the teeth

Use
- Used to obtain a virtual impression of the teeth
- Use software to design the restoration
- Use a specially designed machine to mill the restoration from ceramic blocks

Parts
- A computer with a scanner to obtain the impression intraorally
- Uses a specially designed machine to mill the restoration from ceramic blocks
- Software to obtain the image, design the restoration, and send it to the milling unit
- A specially designed milling unit that uses the directions from the software and cuts the ceramic block to the specifications
- Ceramic blocks in various shades

A. Cerec CAD System
B. Cerec CAM System

Misc.
- Powder normally used to obtain image
- The Cerec scanner uses a blue-light LED camera and the E4D scanner uses a red-light laser to obtain the virtual image.
- The restorations can be milled in the office, which saves the patient from wearing a provisional and coming back for another appointment.
- Auxiliaries can become proficient in designing the restorations to assist the dentist with the procedure.

(*continues*)

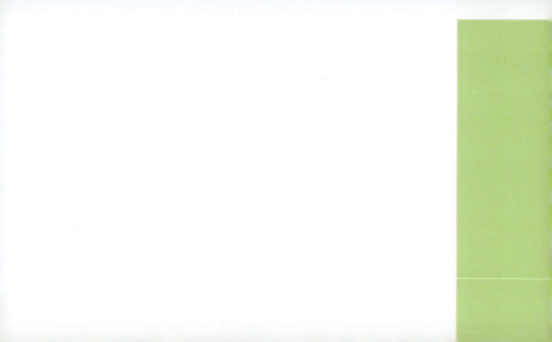

- Some systems will mill bridges and others will only do individual crowns.
- The unit can be moved from room to room for patient access.
- The restoration can be designed, milled, polished, glazed, and seated in one appointment.

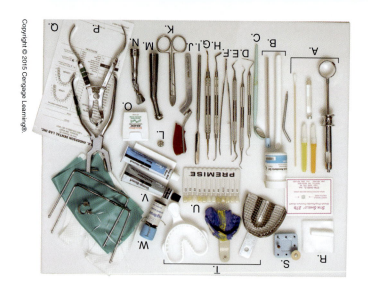

Tray Setup for the Crown Preparation Appointment

| **Use** | This tray is set up when the patient comes into the office for the tooth to be prepared for the restoration. A preliminary (temporary) crown or bridge is normally placed over the prepared tooth until the final restoration can be fabricated unless a CAD/CAM system will be used. |

Parts
- **A.** Anesthetic syringe, carpule, needles, cotton swab, topical anesthetic, and Stik-Shield
- **B.** Three-way syringe tip, high-volume evacuator (HVE) tip, and saliva ejector
- **C.** Mouth mirror and explorer
- **D.** Spoon excavator
- **E.** Curette
- **F.** Cotton pliers
- **G.** Plastic instrument
- **H.** Retraction cord placement instrument
- **I.** Mixing spatula
- **J.** Articulating paper and holder
- **K.** Crown and collar scissors
- **L.** Temporary crown
- **M.** High-speed handpiece

(*continues*)

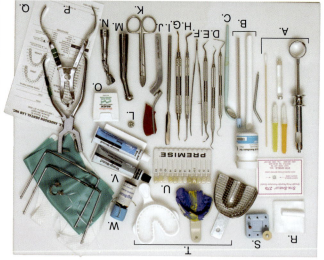

N. Latch-type contra-angle

O. Dental floss

P. Rubber dam placement instruments: punch, forceps, material, face mask, clamp with ligature, and frames

Q. Laboratory prescription

R. Cotton rolls and gauze

S. Miscellaneous burs

T. Alginate and final impression trays

U. Shade guide

V. Temporary bonding material

W. Retraction cord

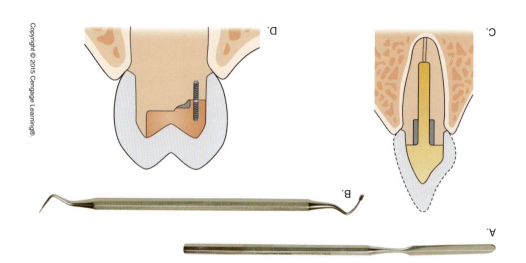

A.

B.

C.

D.

_____ 1. Identify the retention pins.

_____ 2. Identify the core post.

_____ 3. Identify the instrument used for retraction cord placement.

_____ 4. Which instrument is used to gather dental materials for use?

_____ 5. Wrenches or keys for hand placement are used with which instrument?

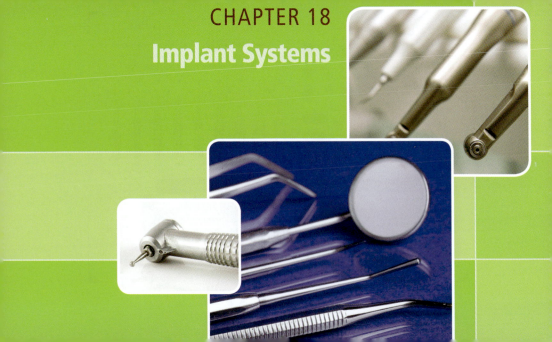

Courtesy of Biocon Dental Implants

Implant System

Use	To surgically place the implant into the jawbone

Parts	An implant system includes the following:

- Pilot drills
- Implant drill stops
- Dental handpiece with no torque and latch-type contra-angle
- Seating tips
- Sulcus reamers
- Latch reamers
- Depth gauge/bone depth plugger
- Surgical mallet
- Paralleling pins
- Guide pin
- Dental implants
- Healing caps

Misc.

- Subperiosteal implants are used on patients whose dentures have failed because the alveolar bone has atrophied (commonly placed on the mandibular).
- Endosteal implants are used to replace a single tooth (placed into the bone and are most commonly used).
- Many different systems are available.

Endosteal Implant

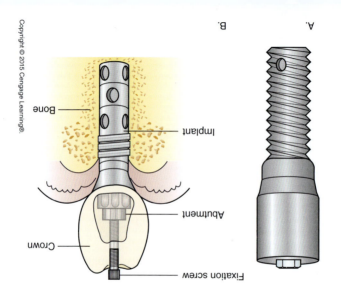

A.

B.

Bone

Implant

Abutment

Crown

Fixation screw

Use	To replace a single tooth
Parts	**A.** Endoseal Implant assembled before placement.
	B. Drawing of an implant in the bone after the healing stage. The abutment of the implant is covered with a crown that is held in place by a screw.
Misc.	• Implants are available in a variety of styles and sizes.

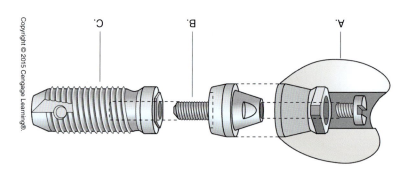

Screw-Retained Implant Prosthesis

A.

B.

C.

| **Use** | • To replace a single tooth |
| | • To replace a tooth and become an abutment for a bridge |

Parts	**A.** Crown covering that screws in to attach the abutment to the prosthesis
	B. Screw to attach the abutment to the implant
	C. Implant that is placed into the bone

| **Misc.** | • Most often, a composite restoration is placed over the screw that attaches the abutment to the prosthesis. |

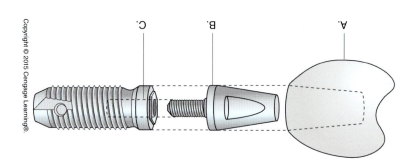

A.

B.

C.

Cement-Retained Implant Prosthesis

Use	• To replace a single tooth
	• To replace a tooth and become an abutment for a bridge
Parts	**A.** Crown cemented onto the abutment
	B. Abutment post that is screwed into the implant
	C. Implant that screws into the bone
Misc.	• Use transitional cement to attach the prosthesis to the abutment.
	• Use in case of problems with the implant

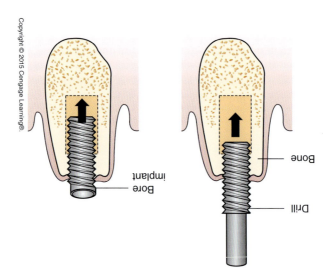

Bore implant

Bone

Drill

Implant Drill

Use	To create a hole in the bone with the precise apical diameter of the dental implant
Parts	Drills in various shapes and sizes that fit into a dental handpiece with a latch attachment that operates without torque
Misc.	• Some drills are color coded according to size. • They have to be kept cool as they are used. • They can only be used a certain number of times, as suggested by the manufacturer. • They must be sterile.

Periodontal Scaler: Implant Scaler

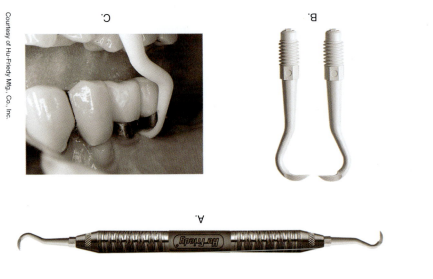

A.

B.

C.

Courtesy of Hu-Friedy Mfg., Co., Inc.

Use	To remove deposits from the dental implants
Parts	**A.** Implant scaler: handle with disposable tips
	B. Disposable scaler tips
	C. Implant scaler positioned around a dental implant
Misc.	• Various designs available to reach around implant
	• Made of materials that will not scratch the titanium implant
	• Some tips are disposable.

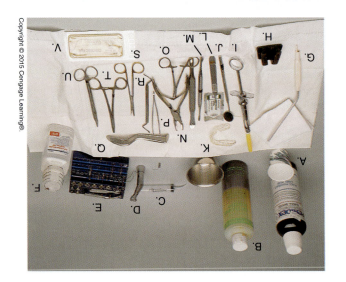

Tray Setup for Dental Implant Surgery

A. Oral rinse with cup
B. Betadine with cup
C. Irrigation syringe
D. Low-speed handpiece
E. Sterile surgical drilling unit/ implant kit
F. Sterile saline solution
G. Surgical high-volume evacuator (HVE) tip on 4 × 4 gauze
H. Bite block
I. Anesthetic setup
J. Mouth mirror

K. Sterile template
L. Scalpel and blade
M. Periosteal elevators
N. Rongeurs
O. Hemostat
P. Tissue forceps
Q. Cheek and tongue retractor
R. Surgical curette
S. Tissue scissors
T. Needle holder
U. Suture scissors
V. Sutures

1. Which instrument is used to scale dental implants?

2. Identify an implant system.

A.

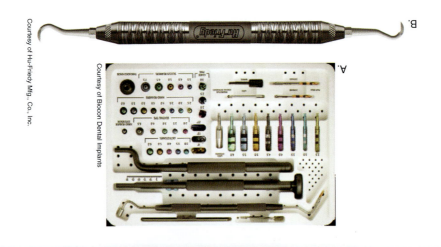

Courtesy of Biocon Dental Implants

B.

Hu-Friedy

Courtesy of Hu-Friedy Mfg., Co., Inc.

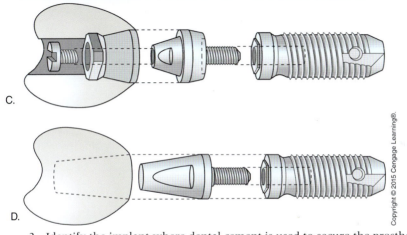

C.

D.

_____ 3. Identify the implant where dental cement is used to secure the prosthesis to the abutment.

_____ 4. Identify the implant where the prosthesis is attached to the abutment with a screw.

Sterilization Equipment

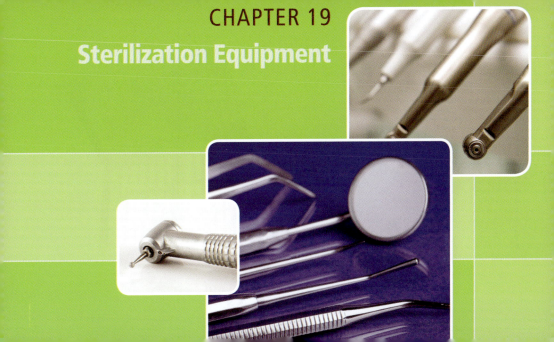

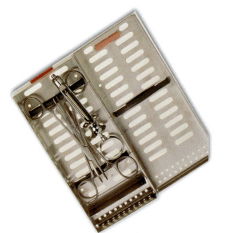

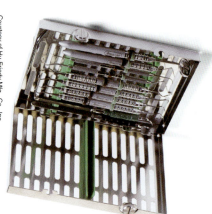

Sterilizing Instrument Cassette

Use	• To contain the instruments while being sterilized and/or stored
	• To use for a tray setup and organization
Parts	• Available in metal or plastic
	• Available in various sizes
	• Many different types of closing devices, but normally hinged on one side
Misc.	• Often instruments are color coded to make it easy to identify which instruments go in which sterilization cassette.
	• Instruments in the cassette can be cleaned in the ultrasonic unit, rinsed, sterilized, and stored in the cassette.

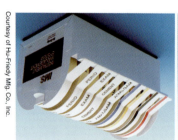
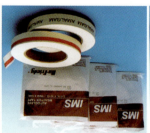
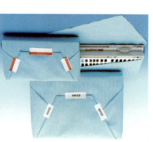

Cassette Wrap and Label System

Use	• To wrap cassette during and after sterilization
	• To use as a tray cover during the procedure
	• To store the sterilized instruments
	• The tape is used to secure the wrap and identify contents.

Parts Wrapping paper, tape, or tape with identification labeling that is used to cover and secure sterilized items or cassettes

Misc.	• Available in a wide range of sizes
	• Tape or labeled tape can be used on sterilization pouches.
	• Tape can be color coded.

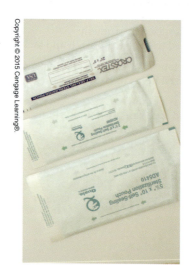

Sterilizing Pouches

Use	• To place instruments in for sterilization
	• Have process indicator dye to verify sterilization
Parts	• Made of clear plastic or paper
	• Sealing strip on the open end
	• Normally have area for labeling
Misc.	• Instruments should be stored in these tightly sealed sterilizing pouches until ready for use.
	• Available in various sizes

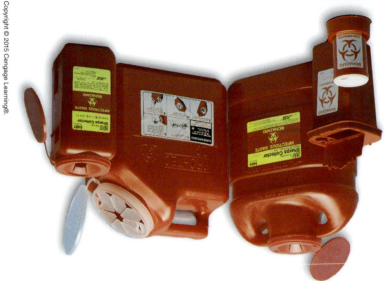

Sharps Container

Use	To contain contaminated sharps, blades, wires, and needles
Parts	• Leak-proof container normally red in color
	• Puncture resistant
	• Labeled
Misc.	• Broken glass, anesthetic capsules, and orthodontic wires can also be placed in the sharps container.
	• When sharps disposal containers are full, they are sealed, sterilized using an autoclave if possible, and sent to an outside biohazard agency for safe disposal.
	• Must be labeled according to Occupational Safety and Health Administration (OSHA) standards (biohazard).
	• Available in different shapes and sizes

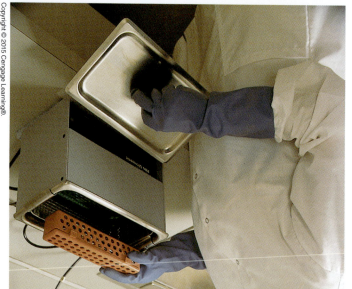

Ultrasonic Unit

Use	• To clean and remove debris from dental instruments and burs
	• Used in place of hand scrubbing the instruments
Parts	• Basket
	• Ultrasonic cleaning device
	• Lid
Misc.	• The ultrasonic cleaning unit significantly reduces the high risk of infection to the dental assistant.
	• It uses sound waves that travel through glass and metal and a special solution to clean the debris from the instruments.
	• This process takes 3 to 10 minutes to complete. During this time, the bubbles implode and produce a cleaning effect on anything within the solution.
	• After cleaning is complete, the instruments are rinsed thoroughly and dried and sterilized.
	• Can be on top of the counter or seated into the counter.
	• Units are available that appear similar to a dishwasher to handle large trays and a number of trays at one time.

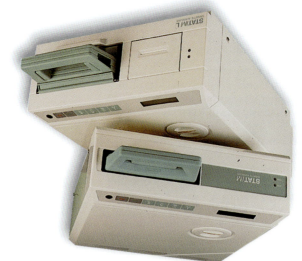

Courtesy of Sci-Can

Use	Quickly sterilizes instruments with steam under pressure
Parts	• Steam sterilizing unit • It uses a hinged cassette that is closed and inserted correctly into the sterilizing unit.
Misc.	• Sterilizes instruments at 270°F • Time: 3 minutes for unwrapped instruments • Time: 15 minutes for wrapped instruments • Easily monitored for accuracy • Requires distilled water • May corrode instruments • Not for use with many plastics • Various styles and sizes available

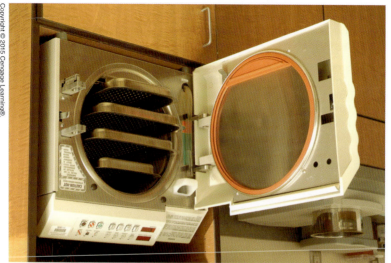

Sterilizer: Steam Autoclave

Use Sterilizes instruments using steam under pressure

Parts Sterilization unit with closing door

Misc.
- Sterilizes instruments at 250°F
- Time: 15 minutes for wrapped instruments/cassettes
- Easily monitored for accuracy
- Requires distilled water
- May corrode instruments
- Various styles and sizes available

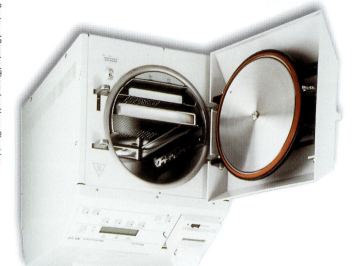

Sterilizer: Chemiclave

Use	Sterilizes instruments using chemical vapor under pressure
Parts	Chemical vapor sterilizing unit with door and pressure chamber
Misc.	

- Sterilizes instruments at 270°F
- Time: 20 minutes for wrapped or unwrapped instruments
- Easily monitored
- Requires proper ventilation
- Requires special chemical solution
- Various types and sizes available

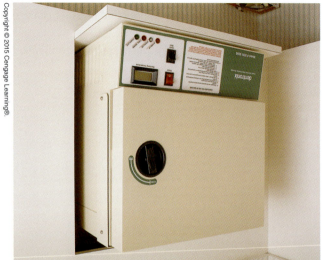

Sterilizer: Dry Heat

Use	Sterilizes instruments using dry heat
Parts	Sterilizing unit with door closure
Misc.	

- Sterilizes instruments at 340°F
- Time: 1 hour for wrapped or unwrapped instruments
- Easily monitored
- Limited rust or corrosion of instruments
- Not for use with plastic/paper
- A dry heat unit that uses forced air is available; this sterilizes in 6–12 minutes.
- Various types and sizes available

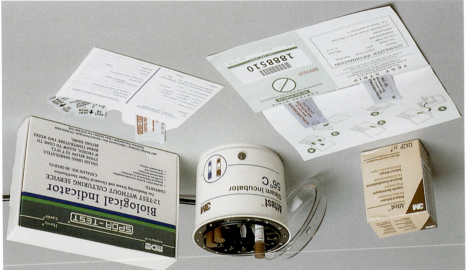

Biological Monitors

Use	Commercially prepared monitors to assess that sterilization has occurred
Parts	Supplied as paper strips or sealed glass ampules of bacterial endospores
Misc.	<ul><li>Placed in the sterilizer along with the instrument load</li><li>When the cycle is complete, the spores are cultured to determine if any have survived.</li><li>The culture can be completed in a dental office if incubators are available for culturing.</li><li>Many are sent out for incubation and a report is returned to the office.</li></ul>

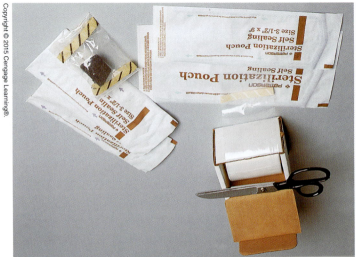

Process/Dosage Indicators

Use	• Process indicators identify whether the packages have been exposed to heat but do not indicate that sterilization has taken place. • Dosage indicators identify if the correct conditions were present for sterilization to take place.
Parts	• Process indicators are normally heat-sensitive tapes or inks printed on packaging materials. • Dosage indicators are dyes placed in the sterilization packing that change color when exposed to dry heat, chemical vapor, or steam for a specific amount of time. • Heat-sensitive tapes or inks are printed on packaging materials.
Misc.	• Process and dosage indicators should also be used with biological monitors.

A.

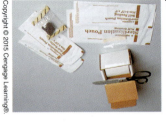

B.

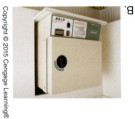

C.

Courtesy of Barnstead/
Thermolyne Harvey Chemiclave

D.

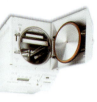

E.

_____ 1. Which sterilizer is the dry heat sterilizer that sterilizes at 340 degrees?
_____ 2. Which sterilizer is the steam autoclave that sterilizes at 250 degrees?
_____ 3. Which sterilizer requires a special chemical solution and proper ventilation?
_____ 4. Which monitor assesses that sterilization has occurred?
_____ 5. Which monitor identifies whether the packages have been exposed to heat?

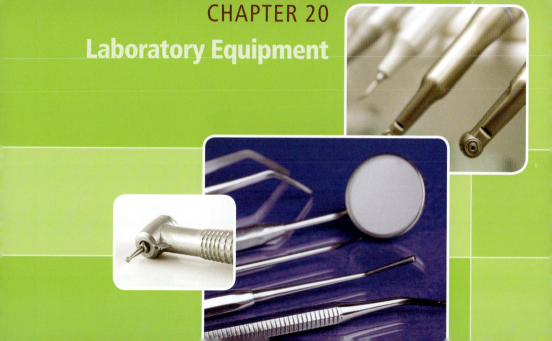

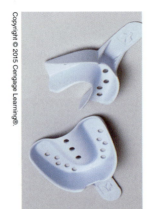

Copyright © 2015 Cengage Learning®.

Disposable Anterior, Posterior, Quadrant, and Full-Arch Trays

Use	• To hold various types of impression materials
	• To carry impression material into the patient's mouth to obtain an accurate impression
Parts	• Perforated trays made of plastic with handles
	• Anterior, full maxillary and mandibular, and quadrant styles
Misc.	• Various sizes that are color coded
	• May be disposable or cold sterilized
	• Can be molded and trimmed if necessary
	• Holes and perforations aid in locking/holding of materials.

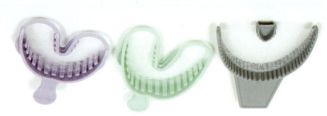

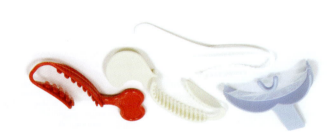

Triple Trays/Bite Registration Trays

Use	• To take a dual-arch impression at one time (using one tray)
	• To take final impressions for crown and bridges and bite registration
	• To take bite registrations for crown and bridge procedures simultaneously while taking the maxillary and mandibular impression (dual-arch-impression technique)
Parts	• Plastic frame with loose webbing to hold impression in tray
	• Thin mesh in the middle of the tray
	• Plastic handle attached
Misc.	• Various sizes and designs for anterior, full-arch, or quadrant impression
	• Disposable
	• Used with various types of final and bite impression materials

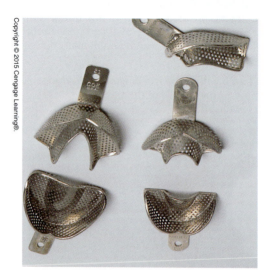

Metal Perforated Trays

Use	To take a dual-arch impression and bite at one time (using one tray) for final impression for crowns, bridges, and bite registration

Parts
- Perforated metal tray with rim
- Handle attached to tray

Misc.
- Various sizes and designs for anterior, full-arch, or quadrant impression
- Sterilized

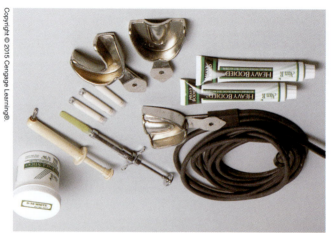

Water-Cooled Trays

Use	To take impressions using reversible hydrocolloid materials and techniques

Parts
- Metal-rimmed tray with locking rim and handle with two tubes
- Comes in full-arch maxillary, mandibular, anterior, and quadrant styles
- Dual hose with two working ends, one end with two attaching areas to the end of the tray and the other end with two attaching areas to the water inlet and the vacuum system outlet on the dental unit

Misc.
- Trays are sterilized.
- Used with reversible hydrocolloid material only
- Connect the hoses to the tray before connecting to a water source.

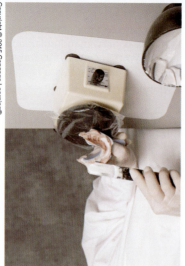

Dental Vibrator

Use	To vibrate materials such as plaster or stone to remove air.
Parts	• Small motor topped with a rubber platform work surface
	• Three speed controls
	• Some come with rubber-cup suction feet to secure the vibrator to the counter.
Misc.	• The rubber platform surface is often covered with a paper towel or plastic to aid in easy clean-up.

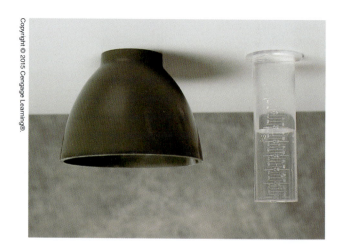

Flex Mixing Bowls

| **Use** | • To mix materials such as alginate and/or gypsum products |
| | • Provide flexibility when mixing materials |

Parts Various sizes of rubber, flexible bowls with a firm bottom

Misc.
- Available in various colors
- Easy to hold and turn in hand while mixing
- Some come with disposable liners.
- Easy to clean after use

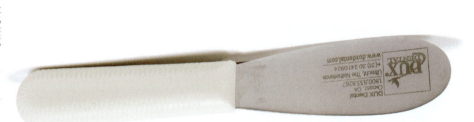

Laboratory Spatula

Use	<ul><li>To mix materials in a flexible bowl</li><li>To mix materials on a paper pad such as a periodontal dressing and/or impression materials</li></ul>
Parts	<ul><li>Blade with handle</li><li>Blades are plastic or stainless steel.</li><li>Handles are plastic, wood, or metal.</li></ul>
Misc.	<ul><li>Various sizes and styles</li><li>Usually 7 1/2 inches long</li><li>Available in a variety of colors</li><li>Some are sterilized.</li></ul>

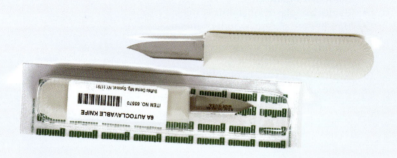

Laboratory Knife

| **Use** | • To trim excess materials from models |
| | • To separate models from impression tray and material |

| **Parts** | Wooden handle with stainless steel knife blade or autoclavable handle and stainless steel knife blade |

| **Misc.** | • Available in different styles with curved or straight blades |
| | • Various sizes available |

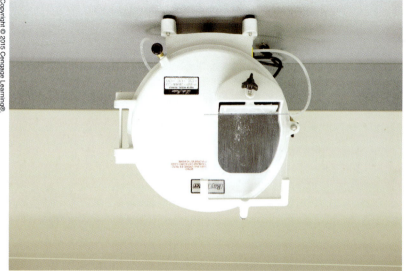

Model Trimmer

Use	• To trim models of extra plaster or stone • To remove excess gypsum material and trim for diagnostic or orthodontic presentation
Parts	• Heavy cast unit with motor • Cutting or grinding wheel • Working table • Water spray and connection • Splash shield
Misc.	• Available in a variety of styles, including a unit with dual grinding wheels • The working table is adjustable to create the angles needed. • The wheels may be reversible. • Water sprays on the wheel to reduce the heat, keep the dust down, and assist in keeping the wheel clean. • Units are usually secured to a table or counter near a water source.

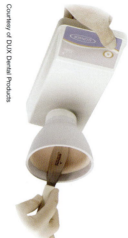

Courtesy of DUX Dental Products

Alginator

Use	To provide a bubble-free, smooth mix of alginate (irreversible hydrocolloid) material
Parts	Motorized unit with controls and pad for flexible mixing bowl
Misc.	• Small portable design that is easy to move from room to room • Bowl rotates to mix alginate and water together while using a spatula • Easy-to-clean bowls that come in different sizes

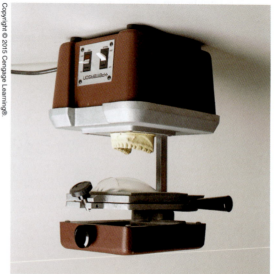

Vacuum Former

Use	• To make custom trays for final impressions
	• To make whitening trays to be used with whitening materials and techniques
	• To fabricate mouth guards, night guards, and splints

Parts
- Unit with heating element and vacuum adapter
- Adjustable arm with heating element and frame to hold sheets under heating unit
- Vacuum table with holes where model is placed
- Controls on the base

Misc.
- Various types of vacuum forming materials are available in different thicknesses.
- Some units have a gasket that needs to be changed to keep a tight seal.
- Once materials are heated, the arm is dropped and the vacuum is turned on to suck the materials tightly to the models.
- Models are wet to prevent small air bubbles.

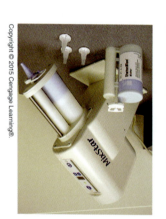

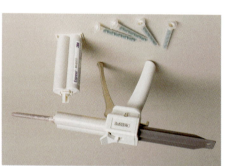

Cartridge-Dispensing Guns and Automixer

Use	• To dispense a variety of dental materials
	• To mix a variety of dental materials
	• To place mixed dental materials

Use
- To dispense a variety of dental materials
- To mix a variety of dental materials
- To place mixed dental materials

Parts
- The cartridge-dispensing gun has a pressure rod and an area for the cartridge to be inserted and secured. Pressure is applied to the trigger handle to mix and dispense materials.
- The automixer unit has brackets to hold cartridges of catalyst and base material; it also has disposable tips, unit controls with on and off, and a locking area for tips.

Misc.
- Used with cartridges of various impression materials, such as polysulfide, vinyl polysiloxane, and polyether
- Used to mix (bite registration, temporary/provisional materials)
- Mixing tips are color coded to indicate various sizes and lengths.
- The tips match the material cartridges they are used with.
- Various styles of automixers available
- The automixer can mix tray material, syringe material, or an alginate substitute material.

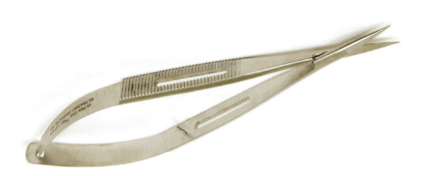

Use	To trim soft tray materials such as whitening trays
Parts	Curved locking handles with sharp pointed blades on working end; lightweight
Misc.	<ul><li>Allow easy manipulation of contours of gingival margin and embrasures</li><li>Sharp at cutting tips</li></ul>

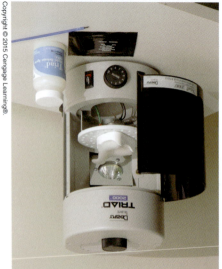

Triad® System

Use	To cure light-sensitive acrylic tray materials
Parts	• A cylinder-shaped heating unit with a wraparound dark window
	• A tray area on which to place model with materials
	• Controls
Misc.	• Used with air barrier coating material, model release agent, BLC bonding agent, modeling tool, and brushes
	• The setting time is controlled by the operator.
	• The light source initiates polymerization.

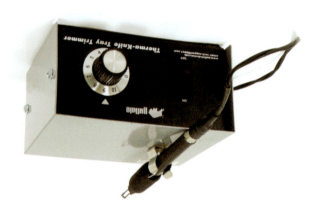

Soft Tray Trimming Devices

Use	• To trim soft tray materials such as whitening trays
	• To trim and contour denture relines, soft night guards, and sports mouth guards
Parts	• Heating unit with adjustable heat settings
	• Handpiece-style handle with curved, double-edged tip that is attached by a cord to the unit
	• Comes with bracket on the unit to hold the knife handle
Misc.	• Easy to use for cutting and trimming gingival margins
	• Used with various tray materials
	• Can be used with materials on the models to prevent distortion
	• Can be used interproximally

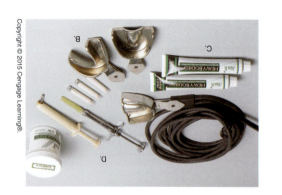

B.

C.

D.

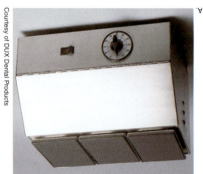

A.

Hydrocolloid Unit

Use	• To prepare, store, and temper hydrocolloid materials used to take a hydrocolloid final impression on crown and bridge procedures
	• To boil hydrocolloid impression materials to convert solid form to liquefied form
	• To store materials once boiled before being tempered and to hold syringe hydrocolloid materials until used
	• To temper hydrocolloid tray materials before placing into the patient's mouth
Parts	**A.** Three-compartment electric unit
	• Tank for converting/boiling materials (212°F/100°C)
	• Tank for storage (150°F/65.5°C)
	• Tank to temper materials before placing them into the patient's mouth (110°F/43°C)
	• The unit has a timer.
	B. Water-cooled trays are used with this system.
	C. Hydrocolloid materials come in tubes for tray impressions and cartridges for dispensing syringes
Misc.	• Materials can be left in the storage compartment for long periods of time so they can be prepared in the morning and be ready for late-afternoon impressions. (*continues*)

- Tray hydrocolloid materials are boiled for 10 minutes and then placed in storage. When ready to use, tray materials are placed in water-cooled trays and then into a tempering bath (tank) for 3–5 minutes.

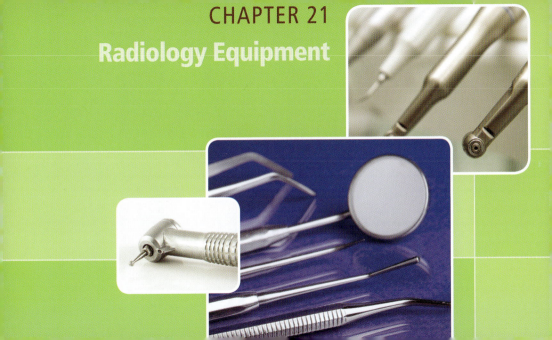

CHAPTER 21

Radiology Equipment

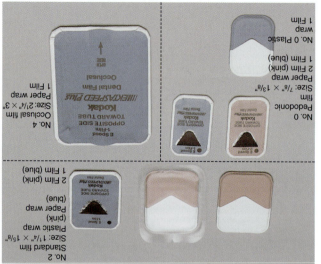

No. 2
Standard film
Size: 1¹/₄" × 1⁵/₈"
Plastic wrap
(pink)
Paper wrap
(blue)
2 Film (pink)   1 Film (blue)

No. 4
Occlusal film
Size: 2¹/₄" × 3"
Paper wrap   1 Film
Occlusal

No. 0
Pedodonic
film
Size: ⁷/₈" × 1³/₈"
Paper wrap
2 Film (pink)
1 Film (blue)

No. 0 Plastic
wrap
1 Film

Intraoral Film Sizes

Use

Offers different sizes of film needed for the correct radiograph

Parts

Film Size	Description/Use
No. 0	Child size
No. 1	Narrow anterior film size
No. 2	Adult size
No. 3	Long bite-wing film size
No. 4	Occlusal film size

Misc.

- Films packets are available with barriers, or barriers may be purchased separately.
- Films are used to take adult and pedodontic exposures—periapical, occlusal, and bite-wing exposures.
- Packaging color and numbering may differ from manufacturer to manufacturer.

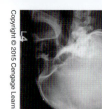

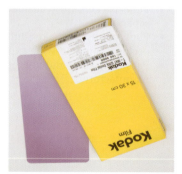

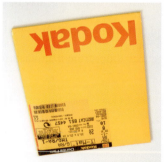

Use	To record extraoral structures such as the teeth and surrounding bone onto the film
Parts	Dental extraoral film held between two screens in a cassette
Misc.	• Different extraoral machines require different types of cassettes to hold the film.
	• Extraoral films can be the panoramic type, which shows the maxillary and mandibular and surrounding tissues on one film, or the cephalometric type, which shows a facial profile that includes the bone, teeth, and soft tissue.
	• Extraoral films must be loaded and unloaded into the cassette under safe light conditions.
	• Some machines have labeling devices to identify patient name and the date the film was exposed.

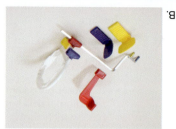

B.

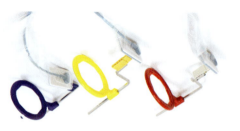

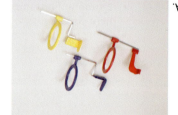

A.

X-ray Film Holder—XCP (X-ray Film Holder with One Ring and Arm Positioning System)

Use	To hold and position x-ray film in patient's mouth and place the position indicator device (PID) while exposing a radiograph; available in anterior, posterior, and bite-wing bite blocks
Parts	**A.** Three each of plastic colored rings, metal arms, and color-coordinated plastic bite blocks
	B. One multi-ring metal arm and three plastic bite blocks
Misc.	• Normally, the red ring and bite block are used for bite-wings.
	• Normally, the blue ring and bite block are used for the anterior.
	• Normally, the yellow ring and bite block are used for the posterior.
	• The XCP is used with the paralleling exposure technique.
	• Digital film holders allow for the cord and have an attachment area.
	• Sterilized
	• The XCP has brand-specific sensor holders that ensure coordination with specific manufacturer equipment.

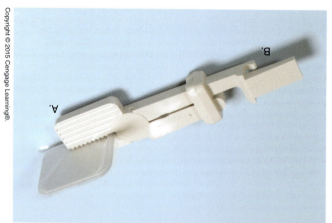

X-ray Film Holder—Snap-a-Ray

Use	To hold and position x-ray film in patient's mouth while exposing a radiograph
Parts	Double ended:

A. The gripping end holds and positions film for posterior teeth and has a biting surface to stabilize the film and holder in the mouth.

B. The end that allows for film to slide in is used on the anterior teeth.

Misc.	

- Sometimes referred to as an EeZee-Grip holder
- Sterilized
- The anterior or posterior can use either size #1 or size #2.
- Can hold either film or phosphor plates securely without damaging them
- The cushioned bite area is good for patient comfort.

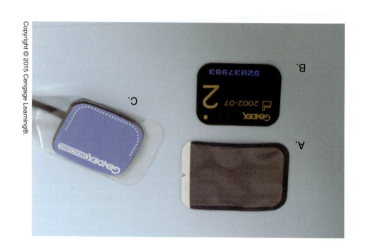

Digital Sensor

| **Use** | • It is an electronic or specially coated plate that is positioned in the mouth and then exposed to radiation. |
| | • It takes the place of traditional x-ray film. |

Parts
- **A.** Barrier
- **B.** Imaging plate
- **C.** Direct digital sensor

Misc.
- Direct digital imaging is where the sensor is placed in the mouth and the image is produced on the surface of the sensor, digitized, and then transmitted to the computer.
- Indirect digital imaging systems convert traditional film x-rays to digital images, which are then viewed and stored in the computer. This system requires that a scanner be used to read the radiographs prior to being transferred to the computer.

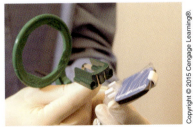

Copyright © 2015 Cengage Learning®.

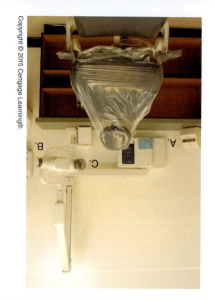

A.

B.

C.

X-ray Unit

Use	To take dental x-rays
Parts	**A.** The control panel has the on/off switch and is where the exposure time is located. It may have adjustments for kilovoltage, milliamperage, radiograph to be taken, and child or adult choices.
	B. Tube head where the x-ray tube is located
	C. Cone or position indicating device (PID) that directs the radiation
Misc.	• Numerous x-ray units are available, each with its own configuration.
	• The operating button is located outside of the room where the x-ray unit is located.

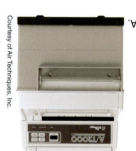

A.

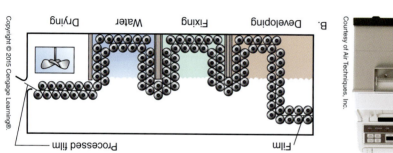

B.

Drying | Water | Fixing | Developing

Film

Processed film

Use	To automatically process exposed radiographs
Parts	**A.** Automatic film processor
	B. Drawing of the inside of a typical automatic film processor
Misc.	• Available with daylight loaders, which allow loading the exposed film in light conditions
	• Proper levels of the chemicals must be maintained to ensure correct processing.
	• The unit must be turned on prior to processing exposed radiographs to allow the chemicals to be heated to the correct temperatures.
	• The film is developed, fixed, washed, dried, and ready to mount within 5 minutes.
	• The developing and fixing solutions used with the unit are different from manual developing and fixing solutions.
	• The unit must be cleaned and maintained properly.
	• Follow the manufacturer's directions.

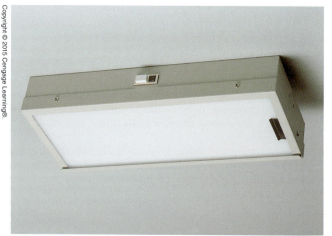

X-ray View Box

Use	To view/read traditional radiographs
Parts	Small cabinet with bright light covered by a flat frosted surface; has a clip to hold the x-rays and an on/off switch
Misc.	• Units may be placed on a counter or mounted on a wall, in a cabinet, or in a dental unit.
	• X-rays are placed on the frosted surface with the raised dot in the convex position so they can be read as if the dentist is looking into the patient's mouth.
	• There are many styles of view boxes available.
	• View boxes are found in each treatment room and also in the x-ray processing area.

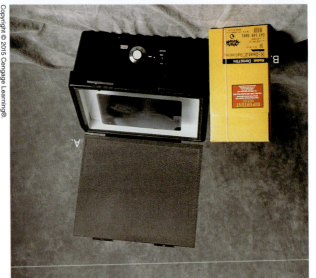

A.

B.

Duplicating Machine

Use	To copy/duplicate x-rays so originals do not have to leave the office
Parts	**A.** Duplicating machine consists of:

A. Duplicating machine consists of:

- Box with a light
- Glass plate on which to place the original x-rays and then the duplicating film
- Controls for exposure time
- Switch to turn the light on when placing original x-rays and then off to place duplicating film
- Latch to secure the lid during exposure

B. Duplicating dental film

- Available in a variety of sizes
- Can be processed manually or with an automatic processor

Misc.

- Duplicating film must be handled under safelight conditions.
- Duplication films are sent with insurance claims and to dental specialty offices when a patient is referred for treatment.
- Duplication films are also used in legal cases, such as malpractice suits or accident cases.

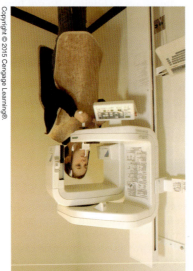

Panoramic X-ray Machine

Use	To expose an x-ray of the entire maxilla and mandible and surrounding tissues in a panoramic view
Parts	• A specialized x-ray machine attached to a column that can be adjusted to the height of the patient • Rotating attachment with an x-ray tube head on one side, a panoramic cassette/cassette holder on the other side, and a head support, bite block, and chin rest in the middle • Controls for patient height adjustment and a digital touchscreen interface for alignment adjustments
Misc.	• Various panoramic machines are available. • Cassettes are specific to the machine. • The patient wears a lead apron without a thyroid collar. • Patients are usually positioned standing up. • Bite blocks are disposable. Head and chin rests are disinfected after each patient. • Laser alignment lights are used to ensure correct positioning of the patient's head. • Some dual-system digital panoramic units will expose temporomandibular joint (TMJ)/sinus modes and perform tomographic imaging. • Panoramic machines that also take cephalometric x-rays and perform 3-D options are also available.

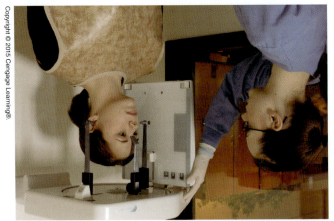

Cephalometric X-ray Machine

Use	• To expose a radiograph of the patient's skeletal structure and profile
	• To aid in orthodontic and oral surgery diagnosis and measurements
Parts	• Specialized x-ray machine attached to a column that is adjustable to the height of the patient
	• Rotating attachment with an x-ray tube head on one side, a cephalometric cassette/cassette holder on the other side, and a head-holding device in the middle
	• Controls for patient height adjustment and a digital touchscreen interface for alignment adjustments
Misc.	• There are two views that can be taken: lateral views and posterior/anterior views.
	• For lateral views, the side of the patient is positioned parallel with the cassette, and earpieces are placed in the patient's ears to align the Frankfort plane.
	• For posterior/anterior views, the patient's head is positioned to face the cassette with the earpieces in place. The x-ray beam is then directed at the occipital bone and perpendicular to the cassette.
	• Cassettes are specific to the manufacturer of the equipment.
	• The patient wears a lead apron without a thyroid collar.
	• Patients are usually positioned standing up.

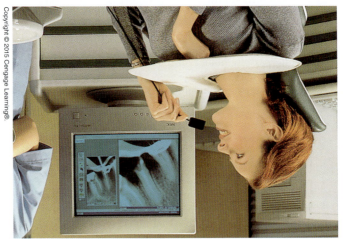

Direct Digital Imaging System

Use	To expose intra- and extraoral radiographs of the patient and display the images on the computer screen

Parts

- Dental x-ray unit, including control panel, timer, arm assembly, and tube head
- Computer monitor and specific digital imaging software
- Sensors or phosphor plates
- Sensor or phosphor plate holders (as described earlier in this chapter)
- Scanner (with indirect imaging systems)
- Barriers

Misc.

- There are several types of digital imaging systems, including direct and indirect methods for obtaining a digital image.
- With the direct imaging systems, the image appears immediately so the dentist can explain findings, diagnoses, and procedures to the patient right at the dental chair.
- With indirect imaging systems, an x-ray is exposed on a phosphor plate, which is then placed on a carousel that is inserted into the scanner to digitize the image to be displayed on the computer screen.
- Both systems have software that allows the digital image to be enhanced, mounted, and stored as part of the patient's records.

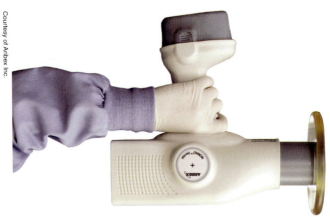

Courtesy of Aribex Inc.

Handheld X-ray Machine

Use	To take/expose x-rays in a variety of dental settings
Parts	Handheld unit includes x-ray tube head, position indicating device (PID) or collimator, shielding, handle with digital control panel, and battery
Misc.	<ul><li>Used in dental offices, military bases, teaching facilities, and clinics, as well as to provide global access to dental care in remote areas</li><li>Settings for adult or child, anterior or posterior x-rays</li><li>Can expose dental film, digital sensors, and phosphor plates</li><li>Units are usually preset at 60 kV and 2 mA.</li><li>The operator is allowed to stay with the patient because the units are handheld.</li></ul>

A.

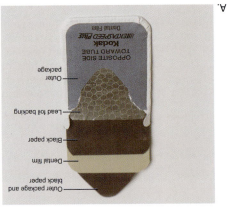

Kodak
|||EKTASPEED *Plus*
Dental Film

OPPOSITE SIDE
TOWARD TUBE

Outer package

Lead foil backing

Black paper

Dental film

Outer package and
black paper

B.

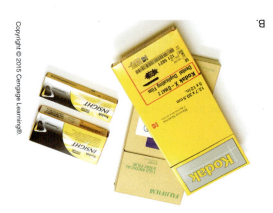

Kodak X-OMAT 2
Dental Duplicating Film
5 x 12 in.
12.7 x 30.5 cm

Kodak

Kodak INSIGHT

Kodak INSIGHT

FUJIFILM

UI MEDICAL X-RAY FILM

Use	To record intraoral structures such as the teeth and surrounding bone onto the film

Parts

A. Film packet
- Outer package and black paper—may be soft plastic or paper
- Dental film—may be a single or double film
- Black paper to protect the film from light
- Lead foil to stop radiation from reaching beyond the film
- Outer package

B. Packaging for x-ray film

C. Comfort Strips
- Comfort pads/strips are available to place over the sharp edges of dental packets.

Misc.
- Film packets are waterproof.
- Films are available with barriers.
- Film speed is indicated on the packets (A–F). The faster-speed film reduces the amount of

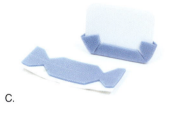

C.

Copyright © 2015 Cengage Learning®.

(continues)

radiation to the patient. Currently, F is the most commonly used and results in much less radiation dosing than D or E.
- Available in double-film packets
- Packaging color and numbering may differ from manufacturer to manufacturer.
- Comfort pads come in a variety of sizes and styles and can be used on intraoral film and digital sensors.

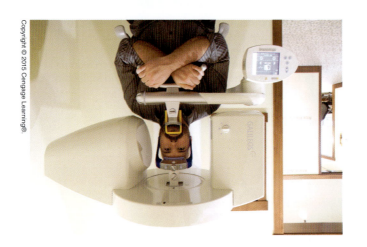

Cone Beam 3-D Imaging System

Use	• To show three-dimensional (3-D) imaging of the patient's mouth, face, and jaw area, including condyles and surrounding structures
	• To produce digital panoramic and celphalometric images, 3-D photos, and computerized tomography (CT) scanning
Parts	• Specialized x-ray machine attached to a column that is adjustable to the height of the patient, with handgrips to stabilize the patient
	• Rotating attachment with two sensors to capture 3-D images and touchscreen controls for capturing areas of interest
	• Laser lights are used for positioning before scanning.
	• 3-D software specific to the individual machine and a computer are required.
Misc.	• Images are used for diagnosis and treatment planning of caries, endodontic procedures, orthodontics, implants, and other oral surgery procedures, and for patient education.
	• Images are also used for nerve mapping, accurate measuring, and determining exact tooth location, as they include views from different angles.
	• Some machines come with 2-D and 3-D capabilities.

(continues)

- Several units are designed to take panoramic and celphalometric x-rays, and perform 3-D options.
- Scans are completed in 8 to 20 seconds.
- Computer software is designed to solve dental problems through perceptive integrations of diagnosis, computer-aided therapy planning, and detailed intraoperative implementation.
- These systems enhance patient understanding of diagnosis and treatment options.

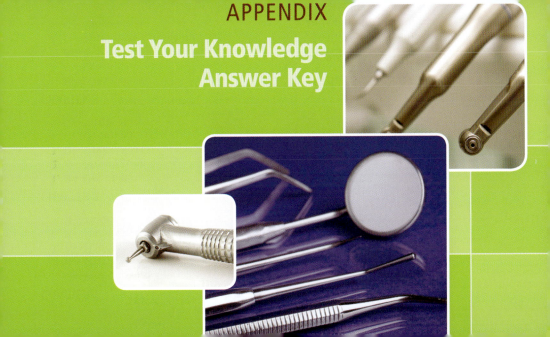

APPENDIX

Test Your Knowledge
Answer Key

CHAPTER 1

1. C—Working end
2. B—Shank
3. A—Handle
4. A—Handle
5. B—Shank

CHAPTER 2

1. B—Dry angle
2. A—Mouth prop
3. D—Utility gloves
4. C—Overglove
5. E—Nitrile gloves

CHAPTER 3

1. B—Forceps
2. E—Expro
3. A—Explorer
4. D—Three-way syringe tip
5. C—Saliva ejector

CHAPTER 4

1. B—Recapping devices
2. D—Local anesthetic; periodontal ligament injection syringe
3. A—Local anesthetic cartridge.
4. C—Local anesthetic; computer-controlled delivery system
5. E—Topical anesthetic

CHAPTER 5

1. D—Anterior or cervical clamp
2. E—Universal mandibular clamp
3. B—Premolar clamp
4. A—Dental dam stamp
5. C—Dental dam forceps

CHAPTER 6

1. A—High-speed handpiece
2. B—Laboratory handpiece

3. C—Fiber-optic high-speed handpiece
4. D—Low-speed handpiece with contra-angle attachment
5. E—Air abrasion handpiece unit

CHAPTER 7

1. A—Plain fissure straight bur
2. D—Inverted cone bur
3. E—Plain fissure cross-cut bur
4. B—Diamond bur
5. C—End-cutting bur

CHAPTER 8

1. C—Hatchet
2. D—Straight chisel
3. B—Excavators
4. E—Hoe
5. A—Angle former

CHAPTER 9

1. A—Dental matrix
2. D—Sectional matrix ring
3. E—Plastic strip matrix
4. B—Plastic filling instrument
5. C—Small balled instrument (dycal instrument)

CHAPTER 10

1. C—Amalgam carriers
2. B—Discoid/Cleoid
3. A—Articulating forceps
4. E—Back-action condenser
5. D—T-ball burnisher

CHAPTER 11

1. C—Applicator
2. A—Well for the composite material
3. B—Composite syringe and cartridge

4. E—Curing light meter
5. D—Curing light

CHAPTER 12

1. B—Glick #1
2. D—Endodontic explorer
3. E—Broaches
4. A—Hedstrom file
5. C—Lentulo spiral

CHAPTER 13

1. B—Surgical curettes
2. C—Surgical bone file
3. E—Chisel and mallet
4. D—#151 mandibular extraction forceps
5. A—#99c maxillary extraction forceps

CHAPTER 14

1. C—Force module-separating pliers (elastic-separating pliers)
2. D—Howe pliers/utility pliers
3. A—Orthodontic bands
4. E—Bird-beak pliers
5. B—Posterior band-removing pliers

CHAPTER 15

1. D—Contouring and crimping pliers
2. A—T-band matrix
3. B—Stainless steel crown kit
4. B—Stainless steel crown kit
5. C—Crown and collar scissors

CHAPTER 16

1. E—Periodontal probes
2. C—Periodontal knives
3. D—Periotomes
4. A—Periodontal rongeurs
5. B—Pocket-marking pliers

CHAPTER 17

1. D—Retention pins
2. C—Core post
3. B—Retraction cord placement instrument
4. A—Cement-mixing spatula
5. C—Core post

CHAPTER 18

1. B—Implant scaler
2. A—Implant System
3. D—Cement retained implant part B
4. C—Screw retained implant part A

CHAPTER 19

1. B—Dry heat sterilizer
2. E—Sterilizer: steam autoclave
3. C—Sterilizer: chemiclave
4. A—Biological monitor
5. D—Process/dosage indicators

Index

Index

Index